Delcia McNeil has practised and taught subtle energy healing since 1983 and is co-Principal of the Rowan School for Healing and Personal Growth. She is a Spectrum and UKCP registered humanistic psychotherapist and a professional massage practitioner. She is a member of a number of professional organisations including the Association for Therapeutic Healers, The National Federation of Spiritual Healers, The Doctor-Healer Network and the International Group for Psychotherapy and Spiritual Healing. She is also an artist who specialises in the abstract painting of energies, thoughts, emotions and sensations. Delcia lives and works both in the Lake District and London, where she has a private practice.

DELCIA McNEIL

Bodywork Therapies for Women

A GUIDE

It is important that you seek appropriate medical advice if you have any symptoms that give you concern. When choosing alternative or complementary practitioners always ensure that they are well-trained and competent.

First published by The Women's Press Ltd, 2000
A member of the Namara Group
34 Great Sutton Street, London EC1V 0LQ

The chakra diagram on page 155 © Jenny Walter 2000

The quotes on page vii are taken from Dianne M Connelly
All Sickness is Home Sickness, (Traditional Acupuncture Institute,
Maryland, USA) and Dr Christiane Northrup *Women's Bodies
Women's Wisdom* (Piatkus Books, London).

British Library Cataloguing-in-Publication Data
A catalogue record for this book is available from the
British Library.

ISBN 0 7043 4569 2

Typeset in Bembo by FiSH Books, London
Printed and bound in Great Britain by Cox & Wyman Ltd,
Reading, Berkshire

This book is dedicated to my dear friend Celia West, in New Zealand, who has truly embraced the meaning of the holistic approach to health and well-being.

Perhaps we shall weave a whole out of our parts. Perhaps we shall wake up as from a deep sleep to possibilities unheard-of.

Dianne M Connelly, *All Sickness is Home Sickness*

No matter what has happened in her life, a woman has the power to change what that experience means to her and thus change her experience, both emotionally and physically. Therein lies her healing.

Dr Christiane Northrup, *Women's Bodies Women's Wisdom*

Contents

Acknowledgements

Creating this book has been a challenging healing journey for me. It could never have been written without the support, knowledge and guidance of many people. A whole network of colleagues and friends, primarily women, has helped me. Many highly skilled and dedicated practitioners and therapists have willingly given their time to read parts of the text and help me compile a resourceful book that I hope is accessible, interesting and lively. To these women I am truly grateful. I also appreciate the contact I have made with women previously unknown to me, and especially to those who contributed their stories. Some of the contributors wanted their names alongside their contributions, others wished to have their first names only, remain anonymous or be acknowledged elsewhere in the book.

There are simply too many to mention here. However, I would like to acknowledge and thank by name the following:

Jill Robinson, Cherith Adams, Dr Sue Morrison, Rosa Shreeves, Jane Gotto, Gillian Rose-Smith, Celia West, Christine Steer, Jan Leake, Jen Altman, Gillian Kelly, Tina Panell, Penny Ingham, Zina Preston, Judy Hargreaves, Della Tysall, Hilary Morgan, Maggie La Tourelle, Anthea Courtenay, Olivea Dewhurst-Maddock, Sheila Adair, Gill Doust, Linda Hall, Susan Willmott, Sarah Craven Webster, Frances Moonwan, Margaret Flavell, Carol Wood, Sue Attrill, Linda Clarke, Marianne Turner, Allison Brown, Silke Ziehl, Bernadette Riley, Sarah Woodruff, Jill Carter, Gill Westland, Mo Strangeman, Mary Hall, Dianne Spencer, Emerald-Jane Turner, Caroline Glading, Susie Roberts, Jenny Walter, Carrie Bates and Lucy Goodison.

A very special thank you to the support from my colleague and friend, Kate Williams, who, particularly in the latter stages of completing the book, has taken more than her share of the responsibility for the work of The Rowan School for Healing and Personal Growth.

I also appreciate several male friends and colleagues who have been helpful and supportive, including Guy Gladstone, Phil Parker and Martin Oakshott. Thank you to John Roberts for his time, energy and photographic skills in helping with the front cover.

Thank you to all my own bodywork therapists past and present, especially Robert Lever, Peter Cockhill, Sue Turner, Sybil Grunberg, Dio Gregory, Ruth France and psychotherapist Maggie McKenzie. Also thank you to my many teachers and trainers over the years, and to my supervisors, Jenny Roth at Spectrum in London and Nigel Wallace in the Lake District.

Thank you to all my clients over the last seventeen years since I have been in private practice and to those I worked with previously when I was a social worker. To all those I have taught over the years – in massage courses during the 1980s and in healing courses since 1983. And a special thank you to the women in the ongoing Women's Therapy and Healing Group that I run. You, my clients and trainees, have taught me more than you will ever know.

Thank you to my family – my sister Sue and my niece Laura, both of whom are in the caring professions, involved with bodywork therapies and contributed to the book with their own stories; to my mother, Marjorie, for teaching me how to be organised, thoughtful and conscientious; and to my father, Fred, for teaching me how to laugh and be witty, to be tolerant and accepting.

A special thank you to Charlotte Cole, my editor at The Women's Press, who I have found to be patient, kind and highly skilled at her job, and to Essie Cousins and the whole Women's Press team.

Finally, my thanks and love go to my husband, Russell, for never complaining when I lost my cool, for all the dinners he has cooked me over the last two and a half years, for his steadying influence, patience, love, healing skills and delightful sense of humour. Apart from supporting me so much personally, his excellent professional skills as a homeopath and fellow therapist, as well as his exceptional command of the English language, have made him a truly supportive friend and colleague.

Some of the therapies I have training in, several I have experienced for myself. However, many were little known or unknown to me before I set out. I have tried to do justice to each of the therapies, to give as much accurate and useful information as possible within the space available. I take full responsibility for any oversights, omissions or inaccuracies and apologise for these in advance.

Introduction

What are bodywork therapies and how can they help you?

Bodywork therapies are a wide range of therapies and treatments generally involving techniques of touch administered by a qualified practitioner. They are non-invasive in the sense that, apart from acupuncture, which uses fine needles lightly penetrating the skin, they do not involve puncturing the body in any way. If you are new to these therapies perhaps you have been struggling with a physical problem for some time and conventional medicine has not really worked for you. If you have not been given a medical diagnosis – and it is important that if you are unwell you get checked by your GP first – you may simply be feeling under the weather or constantly tired. Perhaps you are not sleeping well or find it difficult to quieten your busy mind. Then again you may be feeling unhappy, in conflict emotionally, unable to get your life working for you the way you want. You may have thought about trying alternative approaches to your health but are feeling overwhelmed and confused by what seems to be available, not knowing where to start or what might be right for you.

Alternatively you may already be a committed consumer of the holistic approach and have used one or several complementary and alternative therapies (called CAM for short). Or you may be a practitioner or therapist, or interested in training or academically studying CAM. Whatever has moved you to pick up and open this book, I trust you will find what you need to support you in your journey to health and well-being.

Primarily this is a resource book containing a great deal of information; a friendly reference book, I hope.

Decisions about whether to try a particular bodywork therapy, what to expect, and what to hope for can only be made on the basis of sound information. Most women I know, including myself, hear of therapists 'on the grapevine'. Word of mouth often proves the safest way (although nothing is totally guaranteed; one woman's in-depth wonderful massage is another's too heavy, too insensitive one). Some women read up about a particular therapy before trying it. Others, feeling too weak, low in spirits, or desperate, jump in at the deep end and go along to someone they don't know anything about.

Part 1 of this book is a general look at bodywork therapies and related issues. In Chapter 1, I discuss the holistic approach, the vital ways it differs from conventional medicine and the variety of levels on which it can help you: physical, emotional, psychological and spiritual. I then go on to explore the meanings we give to illness and how our attitudes can affect the outcome.

One of the reasons I am fascinated with bodywork therapies is the touch and contact they give. Touch, in itself, can be very healing. In Chapter 4, I try to explain just how important it is. Finally, I outline how best to find a practitioner. There are issues that as women we might want to discuss with a practitioner; we may feel that another woman therapist is the most appropriate for us. I also give ideas on how to budget for treatments.

Part 2 is a comprehensive guide to today's most widely known therapies. You will find these introduced fully at the beginning of each chapter but to help you use this book I have outlined the main groups and how they might help you:

The **massage therapies**, including the use of aromatherapy, involve different methods of touching the skin, muscles and bones of the body primarily to release muscle tension and help the body and mind relax. Among many benefits, it helps to prevent the build-up of chronic tension.

The **manipulation therapies**, including osteopathy and chiropractic, involve techniques that work on the bones, muscles, tendons, tissue, nerves and spinal-column structure of the body. These techniques are excellent for putting back in place vertebrae that are misaligned and causing pain, and supporting the body to gently realign itself. If you have had any kind of physical injuries these therapies are excellent. Other therapies in this chapter include those for dealing with and learning about postural problems, such as the Alexander Technique. Poor posture can lead to a myriad of physical problems, most especially backache.

Zones, meridians and pressure point therapies come next, in which I explain traditional Chinese medicine (TCM, for short) a system that can treat every ailment. As well as acupuncture and shiatsu I have focused on the bodywork treatments that have evolved from TCM concepts and have been combined with Western thinking, such as reflexology, polarity therapy and applied kinesiology. These touch therapies are particularly good for chronic conditions that have not been helped by conventional Western medicine.

The **metaphysical therapies** involve healing of all kinds. These therapies focus on the vibrational energy of the body and mind and can bring about change in the emotional and spiritual experience of a physical condition. This can then change the whole process of physical disease for the better. They involve touch – both on and off the body – and the use of colour, sound and crystals.

★

The **body psychotherapies** chapter explores psychotherapeutic approaches that are focused on what is happening to and within the physical body rather than only on how we think from our heads. Rather than be a recipient of a treatment from the practitioner or therapist, here you are in a much more dynamic relationship with the therapist. These approaches, such as bioenergetics, gestalt and biodynamic psychotherapy, offer ways of becoming more aware of how we are using our bodies and of how we are creating 'dis-ease'.

The **energy movement systems** chapter, which includes yoga, tai chi, chi gung and Dance Movement Therapy, describes different ways in which we can use movement to increase and balance our energy. Through movement we release tension and keep the structure of the body fit. The importance of physical exercise for good health cannot be overemphasised.

The **convergence therapies** form the final chapter; some therapies simply defy categorisation because they combine aspects of two or often more types. Here I have included some that are newer to the UK, such as the Rosen Method, Zero Balancing and the Trager® Approach. These are light-touch therapies that tend to work on the interface of physical structure, metaphysics and a person's emotional process. They are good for helping us reach optimal health and a feeling of balance and wholeness.

One of the main challenges in writing this book has been to draw boundaries around the information that is available. The definition of bodywork is extremely wide. It could refer to anything that supports the functioning of the human body and mind. There simply has not been room for all the bodywork therapies that exist — and will exist — by the time of publication. The field of bodywork therapies is confusing. In part this is due to the fact that many of the systems and techniques have been 'spawned' and are combinations of a number of related therapies. In addition new therapies are being developed all the time, as expertise and conceptual knowledge becomes more and more sophisticated. Therapists themselves differ in how they think and feel their therapy should be described. To some degree the way I have grouped the therapies is arbitrary; however this kind of differentiation is needed in order to recognise what might be most helpful for what condition, and what may be the most suitable choice.

Most of the therapies can help with practically any kind of condition. All of them share the effect of release from chronic tension, help with pain relief, increased self-awareness, greater ability to relax leading to physical and psychological well-being, possibility of renewed energy and a clearer mind. As all the therapies are concerned with reducing stress, I believe this is one of the major reasons why they have become so popular at this time. The pace and demands of life today are taking their toll on our physical bodies and our emotions. It is becoming essential for people to be able to take an hour or so for themselves regularly to receive a bodywork therapy that slows them down, helps them feel nourished and allows the body time to recharge itself and let go of accumulated strains and stresses.

Where I have thought it would be helpful, I have listed benefits of particular therapies. Where these are not listed it does not, of course, mean that the therapies are not beneficial. Here it seemed more appropriate to describe the value of the therapies within the text. And, of course, you can use the index. In some ways the lists of physical benefits are arbitrary, as practically all of the therapies can help in some way or other with all problems.

I have also indicated contraindications, limitations or possible dangers of therapies throughout the text. Where none are mentioned it is because at present there are none known. I feel it is important to add that none of these therapies carry the dangers of chemical drugs or surgery.

I have excluded, excellent though they are, therapies that involve taking in substances by mouth of some kind, ie homoeopathy, Chinese herbalism, medical herbalism, Ayurvedic medicine (Indian traditional medicine), vitamin and mineral supplement programmes, general nutrition and specialised diets, or flower essences. However, as alternative and complementary therapies, these are important to know about, so I have given definitions of them in Appendix II.

You will find that I interchange the use of the words 'practitioner' and 'therapist'. Practitioner tends to imply a more structured, hands-on approach and therapist is more to do with the process a person goes through in order to heal. A psycho-therapist is rarely called a practitioner, although they do run 'a practice'. In some sections neither is appropriate, eg someone is a teacher of the Alexander Technique, not a practitioner or therapist. Medically speaking, the word therapy refers to the treatment of disease. However, it can also refer to a healing art.

Self-help

Built in to the philosophies of CAM is the belief that we can always help ourselves in some way, no matter how chronic our condition may be. It views the individual as the primary mover in whatever happens. Self-help is integral to the majority of bodywork therapies, so I would advise you to explore further those therapies that really attract you. Where possible, I have given some self-help ideas in the text. Because of limitations of space these really are 'tasters' and tend to be general and straightforward. They have been recommended either by practitioners or by women who have contributed their stories.

The raising of awareness of women's rights in the West in the last thirty years has depended upon women themselves networking, passing information on and sharing experiences. This has certainly happened within the field of alternative and complementary therapies, and I would suggest that CAM's rapid growth, primarily through women, is a direct outcome of women taking more control of their lives. Immediately you are able to do something that will help yourself, the nature of your condition changes. You are no longer a passive victim. You may be a genuine victim, because much of what is happening is not under your direct control, but once a level of personal responsibility is embraced then you can live differently.

Being constantly vigilant to what our bodies need and using self-help techniques give us a means of maintenance and prevention. We tend to know much more about our own bodies than we think we do. We don't have to be academics to understand how our body works and how to look after it.

Women's experiences

An important part of this book is the voices of women, contributions from women who have been willing to share their experiences. Unfortunately, it has not been possible to include a contribution for every therapy described as space would not permit it. Some women wanted to have their names alongside their contribution; others chose to remain anonymous and so I have given them pseudonyms.

It is important to point out that the contents of their stories are the views of the individual contributors. Although they have been selected to help illustrate the main text, they are unique experiences and opinions. I feel it would be unwise to make sweeping generalisations about specific therapies or therapists based solely on these stories.

As I have gathered together these contributions, I have been struck by the fact that many of the contributors have tried a number of different therapies either consecutively or concurrently, creating a personal package for themselves. The commitment to taking responsibility for the maintenance of their own health also comes over strongly.

My experience

Many of the therapies in this book have been paramount in helping me to find my way psychologically and spiritually, as well as to recover from physical pain. Writing about them has been a furthering of my own healing process, and so I invite you to join me in discovering what is possible for you.

As a young woman, in the early 1970s and in my early twenties, I had an eating disorder. I didn't know it was a 'disorder' and it was years later that what I was doing to myself was given a medical name: a diagnosis of bulimia nervosa. I also experienced night-terrors that began at puberty and which, although lessened, remain with me. The reasons for my own difficulties are complex and possibly go back a long way, maybe to the first weeks of my life when my mother suffered postnatal depression. As a young woman my sense of myself was very poor. I didn't experience 'living my life'; my 'life lived me'. I had a young, disastrous marriage and in 1975 at the age of twenty-six, following divorce, became suicidally depressed. I was by then a qualified social worker and was fortunate enough to have heard about psychotherapy. It took me a while, and a recurrence of depression and suicidal thoughts, but in 1977 I decided that rather than end my life I would make a start on healing myself. I made a commitment to life and was willing to do whatever it took to get better. That year I began to receive psychotherapy, initially through the NHS and later privately.

At the age of thirty I injured my back in a roller-skating accident. I fractured one of the vertebrae of the sacrum at the base of my spine.[1] The physical pain and disability resulting from this accident, and my experience of the significant limitations of conventional medicine, led me into a journey of seeking help for myself through bodywork therapies. I also found my true direction in my working life: to take my love and fascination of working with people into the wide field of bodywork therapies. For the last twenty years this work has been the core of my life. Now, at fifty years old, I view the first thirty or so years of my life as my 'initiation' as a healer. My experiences were my training ground, and for this I am truly grateful. Experiencing severe emotional and physical pain has given me a compassion that I could not have known before. I'm not saying I believe we necessarily have to suffer in order to grow, I just believe that it has helped me sort out my own values about what truly matters in my life: honest and loving connection with myself, others and the world in which I live.

The benefits of alternative and complementary therapies depend on what you are seeking help with, the availability of particular therapies, the nature of the techniques or approach used, and the compatibility between yourself and the therapist you choose. They also depend on your expectations, your willingness to take part in the treatment, and being open to looking at what may need changing in your life. Injury or illness is part of life and sometimes there is no obvious or conscious way we could prevent it. However, much of bodywork is about preventative medicine and maintaining good health. It is also about finding out how your own body works, how unique your own system is, and how much your emotions, thoughts and beliefs affect your physical well-being.

Part One

Bodywork Therapy and the Holistic Approach to Health

Chapter One

The Holistic Approach

What does holism mean?

In its simplest form holism means what it says: 'whole'. The Concise Oxford Dictionary defines 'whole' as 'uninjured, unbroken, intact or undiminished state, not less than, all there is of, entire, complete, with no part removed.' It further defines 'holism' as 'the theory that certain wholes are to be regarded as greater than the sum of their parts: the treating of the whole person including mental and social factors rather than just the symptoms of a disease.'

Holistic medicine is concerned with integrating all aspects of our being: body, emotions, thinking and spirit. It is also concerned with prevention. The American Holistic Medical association defines it as 'a system of health care which emphasises personal responsibility, and fosters a co-operative relationship among all those involved, leading toward optimal attunement of body, mind, emotions and spirit.'

From the holistic perspective there is no separation between our bodies and minds. This approach adds other dimensions to conventional medicine, and sometimes challenges the premises on which modern medicine is based. It is developing fast both within and outside the medical profession. Within, it stems from a response to find new methods of dealing with stress-related, and chronic, degenerative illnesses. Outside the medical profession it reflects a concern from the public about long-term dependency on drugs, and their side-effects. Having said this, a doctor can be holistic and prescribe drugs, and an alternative practitioner can be mechanistic in approach.

Sometimes, as a patient, you may not feel fully heard by your doctor because, if your experience does not fit into the model of conventional medicine, then theoretically it doesn't exist. Your experiences may be referred to as anecdotal and therefore not really valid in a scientific way. This can lead you to feel powerless on top of feeling ill. The doctor may also be feeling anxiety because she or he has, in a way, been set up within this model to be able to explain your physical suffering with medical facts. Dr Christiane Northrup states, 'Science must acknowledge truthfully how much it doesn't know and have room for mystery, miracles and the wisdom of nature'.[1]

How do alternative and complementary therapies differ from conventional medicine?

To me the key difference between these approaches is that of vitalism – life force. Conventional medicine is now embracing holism more, in that lifestyle and general well-being are being taken much more seriously in the management of disease. However, conventional doctors do not accept that energy – the movement of life force throughout the human organism – can be worked with therapeutically.

Conventional medicine is the study of the mechanics of the human body. In this schema, the body is reduced to structural parts, proceeding from organs to tissues, tissues to cells, cells to molecules. The whole is separated into parts in order to discern the nature, proportion and function of each constituent. This means that conventional doctors may see a diseased entity as a faulty component and separate it from the organism as a whole. Then it can either literally be removed or treated in isolation from other organs and tissue parts. Just like the car; if it breaks down you go and have it checked, having new parts if you need them. It is the isolated symptom, or group of symptoms, which is the focus of concern.

Sometimes it is appropriate or essential to remove a diseased part because the whole organism can be exhausted in its endeavours to heal the disease, or because this part seriously threatens the life of the whole organism. Sometimes surgery is the best way to treat or repair the body. Unfortunately, possible alternatives to surgery within alternative and complementary health care are often not known about, not tried or are not available. It is likely that a significant amount of surgery could be avoided.

Appendix I describes some of the major differences between the more orthodox and holistic models of health care.

Why do we have alternative *and* complementary therapies? What's the difference?

Generally speaking, alternative therapies, such as acupuncture (from traditional Chinese medicine (TCM)), homeopathy, medical herbalism and Ayurvedic medicine, are complete systems of medicine in their own right (see Appendix II for short descriptions of all of these). Complementary therapies are those which easily support any orthodox treatment, and are not in direct conflict with the philosophy of conventional medicine. However this does not mean to say that acupuncture, homoeopathy or herbalism cannot work well alongside orthodox medical treatment. This whole area is one of debate.

I find it easier to think of continuums within medicine; many people are trying alternative or complementary therapies before having more 'invasive' medical treatment.

Alternatively, they may try these therapies where orthodox treatment hasn't helped. However, it is vital that people receive orthodox medical treatment when they need it. There are failures and successes in both fields. There is also the rapid pace of development of medical technology, which already means that the NHS cannot resource all that could be possible for people. Therefore the need for alternatives, prevention and maintenance of good health is needed more than ever.

Faith in conventional medicine and extensive use of drugs

Every year in Britain, 1.17 million people – a population the size of Birmingham – are put in a hospital bed as a result of a medical procedure that has gone wrong.[2] Another way of putting this is that there is a one in six chance that if you're in hospital you are there because of a modern medical treatment that hasn't worked or has gone wrong. This is called 'iatrogenesis': medically induced illness.

Although wonderful life-saving procedures take place within our hospitals, our belief in conventional medicine can override the acknowledgement of its dangers. Our faith in medical science is so ingrained that it has become woven into our daily reality. Ted Kaptchuk refers to the assumption that 'current Western science and medicine have a unique handle on truth – all else is superstition.'[3]

Countless women and men are questioning the usefulness of the drugs they are prescribed. Avoiding the overuse of antibiotics is now on the public agenda. We have yet to have an open, public debate about the alternative views on mass immunisation.

Doctors can sometimes minimise the risks of drugs by magnifying the risk of not taking them. But side-effects aren't 'side' effects; they are direct effects. When the right drug in the right dosage works it is obviously positive. But often the symptoms from taking a drug are worse than the original symptom it was taken for. Sometimes it is worth it. Sometimes it isn't. Sometimes there is genuinely no other choice and a drug, with its side-effects, is the best thing available.

If your doctor knows you have not taken what he or she has prescribed they may experience this as a rejection of their expertise. Understandably, the doctor will sometimes feel bound to say 'you have to live with it'. This could be because his or her knowledge about other possibilities is limited or non-existent. Fortunately this is changing. This change is coming from both outside and inside the medical profession; from GPs who are not happy with the amount of prescribing they do and from nurses, physiotherapists and doctors who have gone on CAM courses.

One of the biggest problems with medical drugs is the power of the pharmaceutical companies. The majority of medical research is funded by the very companies who stand to gain by certain results. So these companies pay the researchers' salaries and can often decide whether or not the results get published. It is wise to keep in mind that this industry, in a sense, has a vested interest in ill health: if drug companies found cures, they'd soon be out of business.

We have tended to view medical science as omnipotent, with doctors being major authority figures for both men and women. This leaves doctors with an enormous burden of responsibility. It is no wonder that sometimes doctors experience intolerable stress.

My concern is that, as complementary therapies become more and more popular, the medical profession will insist on being in control of them. Complementary and alternative therapists will be institutionalised and lost within the framework of the medical model, with doctors still having the overall control of decision making and resources. Some doctors already have access to training in other therapies, such as hypnosis or acupuncture, but, unless they completely retrain, they receive much shorter training than the therapists in those fields. Some doctors do choose to retrain completely. However, the public can often put more faith in receiving an alternative therapy from a doctor who has less training and experience, simply because he or she is a doctor. This highlights the power that society invests in the role of the doctor. Alternative and complementary practitioners need to continue to develop a professionalism that earns them equal respect. I believe this will come as solid research into the benefits of these therapies continues to build, and a stronger social and political infrastructure is developed within the alternative and complementary therapy profession.

'Complementary medicines have proliferated dramatically in the United Kingdom (and indeed in other European countries) since the 1970s, the increase in the number of practitioners being matched by an increase in usage by consumers. They are no longer marginal to the total system of health care.'[4]

Integrated medicine

Most of the therapies described in this book are complementary to conventional medicine. You are always advised to seek medical help first. You may not choose to accept the medical treatments, but a medical diagnosis is extremely valuable and the treatment may be absolutely essential or simply just right for you.

It can be possible to fall into the chasm between orthodox medicine and alternative treatment, and this can be frightening. The orthodox treatment may not be working, or may be making things worse, but if you turn to something outside the orthodox system and your doctor doesn't approve, then you jeopardise your relationship with him or her. If you go ahead anyway and then the alternatives don't help either, where does that leave you?

Integration is beginning to take place and I hope that both conventional and complementary and alternative approaches will be formed into a new force within health care, whereby the patient will have many more choices and neither the medical establishment nor the complementary or alternative practitioners will have power over the other. An alternative to integrated medicine could be along 'parallel' medicine. This exists in India, where Ayurvedic, homoeopathic and conventional Western medicine are available to the public separately, with each discipline accepting the others.

Sarah Cant and Ursula Sharma make the point that it is not the body of knowledge — and this is now vast — of alternative and complementary medicine and therapies that will make them socially and politically acceptable but, rather, the recognition from the state and the support of the medical profession.[5] High-level skill and information is not only relatively unknown to the general public, medical professionals and administrators, and politicians, but is also not widely available within our health-care structures.

It is also important to remember that the descriptions in Appendix I are based on generalisations. Not only is much of holism entering the orthodox, but also holism is not adopted by all complementary practitioners.

It can be said that some practitioners use the word holistic very loosely. They may view their particular therapy as the best, or the right, way. The best professionals will tell you about their particular therapy but they will not attempt to push it on you or make any exaggerated claims about what it can do for you (see Chapter 4). They will be honest with you and realistic. All of us have been conditioned into believing in the medical model, so it may take an act of faith to put some confidence back into yourself and into alternative techniques, treatments and theories. It also takes a commitment to gather the information and make choices – both medical and alternative or complementary – from this. This may not be easy, especially when you are unwell.

How did this all come about? Mind and matter; philosophies and health

The philosophy of medical science is based on the premise that reality is located in the tangible structure of matter, which can be measured, quantified and analysed. This actually began with Aristotle's 'empirical materialism' and was rediscovered during the Renaissance (the fourteenth to sixteenth centuries AD). Matter was understood to be fixed and unchanging, therefore 'real'. In the seventeenth century Descartes introduced analytic, reductive reasoning and formed the basis of a new philosophy of science. This became the philosophy of modern medicine. 'All science is certain, evident knowledge. We reject all knowledge which is merely probable and judge that only those things should be believed which are perfectly known and about which there can be no doubts.'[6]

So Descartes set up a firm division between mind and matter: 'There is nothing in the concept of body that belongs to the mind; and nothing in that of mind that belongs to the body.'[7] Isaac Newton then followed, taking this mechanistic view further and outlining the cause-and-effect method of explaining the material universe. The universe is made up of solid objects, called atoms. It is a huge mechanical system running on 'laws of motion'. 'Everything could be described objectively. All physical reactions were seen to have a physical cause, rather like balls colliding on a pool table.'[8] This is the basis of the logic of the scientific method and really remains essentially the same today.

The way the Western scientific method works is to find agreement between experimental and mathematical proof. If this agreement is not found, the physicist will search for another theory until proof is found. This scientific method has led to great inventions such as the harnessing of electricity and the use of subatomic phenomena, such as X-rays and lasers, in medicine. When new phenomena are discovered that cannot be explained by the theories that exist, new experiments are carried out until new proof is found.

However, the phenomenon of electromagnetism in the early nineteenth century could not be described by Newtonian physics, and in 1905 Albert Einstein's Special Theory of Relativity told us that space is not three-dimensional and time is not a separate entity. 'Both are intimately connected and form a four-dimensional continuum, called "space-time".'[9] It is in this fourth dimension that we experience telepathy, synchronicity, time speeding up or slowing down, psychic flashes and inspirations. We tend to invalidate these because we are trying to fit them into a linear, Newtonian view of reality.

Atomic physics presents us with the paradox of light or electromagnetic radiation having a dual nature. This radiation consists of both waves and moving particles.

Subatomic particles, which make up the atom, cannot be pictured as a thing or an object. Quantum mechanics views subatomic particles as 'tendencies to exist' or 'tendencies to happen'. How strong these tendencies are is expressed in terms of probabilities. At the subatomic level mass and energy are interchangeable. Since we are made up of atoms we can say that our thoughts, feelings and physical mass are totally interrelated. 'The whole universe appears as a dynamic web of inseparable energy patterns. The universe is thus defined as a dynamic inseparable whole which always includes the observer in an essential way.'[10] So we are part of an interwoven pattern of light, of dancing energy.

At the moment modern medical practice does not reflect the current understanding of the universe as described by quantum physics. It remains based on a Newtonian view and Newtonian laws of the universe. Our own consciousness – the way we think and perceive – still tends to be rooted in this latter view.

'One of the important lessons I learned was that much of what we think is extraordinary in another place is just the ordinary not understood or experienced'
(Ted Kaptchuk describing his journey to the East in *Chinese Medicine; The Web That Has No Weaver*).

Of course, outside the consciousness of science there are other worlds, too; those of the emotions, of feelings, and of political values. There is always a social and historical context in which any knowledge exists and there is the world of the individual and collective unconscious. The holistic model draws much of its understanding from Eastern philosophy. Within the latter, all things and events perceived by the senses are interrelated, connected, and are but different aspects or manifestations of the same ultimate reality. In Buddhist philosophy 'our tendency to divide the perceived world into individual and separate things and to experience ourselves as isolated egos in this world is seen as an illusion which comes from our measuring and categorising mentality.'[11]

The physical body is viewed as a miraculous piece of material equipment that houses the physical organs that sustain life *and* the person's emotional and psychological make-up. For example, the Chinese physician assesses the patient's specific and general physiological and psychological responses to a disease (see Chapter 7). But a word of warning: just because something is more ancient, spiritual or holistic it is not necessarily more 'true' than Western medicine. What is important is a synthesis, a bringing together of these different ways of thinking.

Bodywork therapies and our health on all levels

I have divided these levels into three: physical, emotional and mental, and spiritual. Bodywork therapies work on all levels, depending on the kind of help sought and the focus of the therapist. All of the therapies described in this book can help with most conditions. It is important to be willing to try out different ones to find which suits you.

The contributions to this book from a wide range of women show that you can use a number of different therapies, sometimes one after the other, sometimes simultaneously. Compatibility is essential here. For example, I find that healing, massage, cranial osteopathy and homoeopathy go really well together. Some alternative systems should not be used at the same time – eg acupuncture and homoeopathy – simply because they are such different approaches. Suitability also includes who the therapist is, as well as the techniques tried. You need to feel comfortable with the therapist. Here is one inspiring story from Bettine Goldberg, who has used CAM throughout her life:

'I am English, aged eighty-five and have a son who is in the "spirit world". My husband passed over twenty-four years ago. I live alone. I have always been very athletic all my life and still swim every day in the unheated water of the Serpentine [London]. Also, since my twenties, I have had a weekly Swedish massage. It is part of a keep-fit approach to life and I find small problems can be dealt with before they become serious. For the last two years I have cut down the Swedish massage to once a fortnight and I go for holistic massage and aromatherapy on the alternate week.

During the war I was introduced to osteopathy and have gained enormous benefit from it throughout my life. Like many tall people, from time to time I have problems with my lower back, but this is instantly cured after manipulation. Down the years there have been other small injuries. My osteopath is also brilliant at cranial osteopathy, and his ex-wife is an acupuncturist and has treated me for various small things. I first experienced acupuncture in Hong Kong, where a Chinese doctor treated a neglected frozen shoulder in one manipulation. Having unblocked it he treated me daily with acupuncture to soothe the nerves.

I do not use conventional medicine if I can avoid it and have a very clever homoeopathic doctor. I am extremely fit, young looking and active with a very full life.'

Physical

Many physical symptoms are the end result of a process that begins weeks, months and even years before the pain or discomfort is felt. When I am suffering all I want is to find the key to making it stop. Many people go to bodywork therapists because they are in pain and their doctor has been unable to help them. Or they are on permanent painkilling drugs and want to find ways of getting relief more naturally. Because relaxation is a key component of most of these therapies there is always a good chance that pain will reduce or go completely.

However, it is important to be realistic and not to get carried away with the claims that some therapists make. Often these claims come about because one or two clients have done very well with a particular therapy. Therapists often train in a therapy that they have found remarkable for themselves. Their natural enthusiasm can then often lead to an expectation that everyone else will get remarkable results, too. But responses vary. We also respond differently at different times.

I know that without a minimum of a monthly massage

treatment it is likely that I will get backache. These treatments not only prevent pain but also keep me in touch with my body and how I am using it. It is much harder to consistently over-extend myself when I am treated by a therapist regularly. So much physical ill health is caused by self-abuse: ignoring the signals the body is giving to stop or rest or take exercise or eat good food.

The kind of physical problems that women seek help with are often to do with our reproductive systems – periods, preg-nancy, childbirth, menopause and ageing. We may suffer from thrush, cystitis, vaginitis, fibroids, ovarian cysts, breast lumps, endometriosis and many other lesser known conditions.

On a more general level we may suffer back pain, migraines, have low energy and have depleted immune systems that may lead to colds, flus and more serious conditions such as ME, MS, Aids, heart disease and cancer. We may turn to bodywork therapists when medical treatments are ineffective, or when we want other help to support us through the medical treatment. We may use bodywork treatments to prevent chronic conditions, to help us maintain good health. We may use them both to help us get better and then to continue to maintain health. We may be so ill that we are using these therapies to help us in our dying.

Also remember that in receiving complementary therapies, you may feel worse before you feel better. This is because sometimes the body needs to go through a process of regain-ing equilibrium so that deeper aches and pains can come to the surface to be healed. Sometimes it is difficult to tell whether ongoing discomfort is such a process or whether a therapy is simply not working. Usually we can feel instinctively that something different is happening and that 'things are moving' in the body, even though we may not feel 'cured'. When we are new to the therapies we are likely to feel anxious when we feel worse. It is uncomfortable to change, and to move from the security of the medical model to 'not knowing' as the body reorganises itself to heal.

People vary as to how long they like to stay with a therapy before giving up. Belief in it working at some point really helps. I needed to do this when I was using osteopathy to recover from my back injury. I was still in pain after a year of treatment, but it was important to look back over that year and see how far I had come in my healing journey.

Psychological and emotional

Loss of touch with our bodies can actually result in loss of touch with reality. When I receive a massage I feel back in touch with myself, as if I needed reminding that I am embodied, that I have a physical limit in the form of my skin. 'Personal identity has substance and structure only insofar as it is based on the reality of bodily feeling.'[12]

Alexander Lowen shows in his book *The Betrayal of the Body*, which is a clinical study of people with schizophrenia, that the feeling of identity arises from a feeling of contact with the body. In schizophrenia there is a complete loss of body contact so that the person doesn't know who she is. She is likely to be aware that she has a body and is oriented in time and space but her actual sense of self or ego is not identified with her body. She 'does not perceive it in an alive way, s(he) feels unrelated to the world and to people. Similarly, his (her) conscious sense of identity is unrelated to the way s(he) feels about him(her)self.'[13] When we are emotionally healthy our image of ourselves agrees with the way we feel and look.

If we are unable to feel through our physicality, through touch and physical sensation, we will have difficulty feeling our emotions. We are likely to become withdrawn and detached from others, or feel we are going through life playing a role. We may only be able to make contact with others through words, not with the whole of our being.

When we do feel more in touch with our bodies we may feel painful and negative emotions that we have been unable to let go of. These take their toll on our physical bodies. Such emotions can include grief, feeling overwhelmed, anxious, fearful, bitter or resentful. However, we also start to feel pleasurable feelings: joy, excitement, and love.

Spiritual

'We touch heaven when we lay our hands on a human body' (Novalis (pen name of Frederich von Hardenberg), 1772).[14]

You really need to experience certain types of bodywork to understand how they can help your spirit or soul. These are aspects of our being that are very difficult to put into words. People often describe receiving certain therapies as feeling held, feeling that they are 'coming home' to the body. They experience a deep peace and relaxation. Sometimes, because of this relaxation, a solution to a problem just comes to mind, or an insight is gained. People often go into a semi-dreamlike state when they are on the treatment couch and feel they are floating. Some feel lighter than they have ever felt, others see beautiful colours or images in their mind's eye. This can be particularly uplifting if you have been stressed out and really caught up in the day-to-day living of the material world.

The body can be viewed as a vehicle for the unconscious mind and so receiving touch that is therapeutic can become a way through to understand our inner emotional and psychic processes in a deeper way. People experience shifts of energy within the body, rather like natural electrical currents, which give a sense of being 'unblocked' or freed up. Afterwards people generally feel more balanced on all levels. However, as mentioned earlier, sometimes the treatment can make you feel worse temporarily, either because the experience has made you stop and really feel your discomfort or exhaustion, or because toxins in the body are being shifted. It is important to talk to your therapist or practitioner if you feel disturbed by a treatment so that she can assess the level at which she is working and can give appropriate advice.

Frances Tyler-Rides' story illustrates how important spirituality can be in reaching and maintaining good health:

'I am a working class, white, English woman aged thirty-three. I have three children and am just leaving a partnership. I am a full time student, part-time volunteer worker, coordinator of a crisis line and sell advertising part-time.

My search for good physical and mental health has led me to complementary medicine. I have found it very helpful and effective when I've had the time to follow it regularly! I suffer from chronic asthma and hormonal disturbances. I am registered disabled but am fortunate that for much of my life these health problems have not dominated my lifestyle, although recently things have changed.

I am open to making lifestyle changes but do find it hard to incorporate them in my daily life, as society does not encourage such 'weirdness' – dairy and gluten-free eating and the use of essential oils, massage, homeopathy and herbalism – as norms.

My experiences within bodywork therapies have been very good, but have not remained in the physical realm. I have found aromatherapy reaches the parts other less holistic methods haven't, and also that spiritual healing, crystal healing and tai chi bring about an awareness of being a part of a whole, vibrant, living being that some would call 'the cosmos'.

I suspect that if humanity could embrace bodywork therapies more, we would hate each other and ourselves less.

In particular, I would recommend aromatherapy, tai chi and yoga for people with breathing problems. Osteopathy is an amazing therapy and achieves equally amazing results, and I would personally recommend it for anything, from whiplash to chronic body damage from violent ex-partners.

In addition, I would like to add how empowering it is to be listened to and treated as an individual instead of a stereotype of womanhood.'

Chapter Two

The Meaning of Illness

How do we give meaning to our experience?

It is fascinating how the meanings we give to our experiences can directly affect the quality of our lives and often the outcome of our illnesses.

Ken Wilber in his book *Grace and Grit* questions both conventional and New Age approaches to illness. He tells the moving and compelling story of his wife Treya's five-year journey through her illness, treatment and final death from cancer. He combines Treya's journals with a wide-ranging commentary exploring the differences between spirituality and religion, psychotherapy and women's spirituality, and approaches to health and illness. He offers us a critique of the many ways in which we attempt to bring meaning to our understanding of illness. 'Men and women are condemned to meaning, condemned to creating values and judgments. It is not enough to know that I have a disease... I also need to know why I have that disease. Why me? What does it mean? What did I do wrong? How did this happen?'.[1] Often this breeds negative judgments about illness – that if we are sick we must be bad.

He goes on to say that the values and meanings given to a particular disease are culturally defined, and he describes several cultural and subcultural ways in which we attempt to do this, all of which I found I could identify with. Here are several:

We may see illness as a punishment for having sinned: the **fundamentalist Christian** view. Or it is a lesson and on some level we are choosing the experience of ill health in order to evolve spiritually: this is the **New Age** view. For example, this is how I gave meaning to my own back injury. I believe I needed to go back to my 'root' (my sacrum) in order to find my right direction in life. Then again, illness can be seen as purely a biophysical disorder caused by factors such as virus, trauma, genetic predisposition or environmental agents that trigger negative physical responses: this is the **medical view**. As Caroline Myss states in the *Anatomy of the Spirit*, 'Conventional medical philosophy considers the patient an innocent – or virtually powerless – victim who has suffered an unprovoked attack.'[2] This is the view held by many people.

There is also a view that illness is the result of 'negative karma'. **Karma** is the spiritual law of cause and effect. Belief in karma has to include a belief in reincarnation and personal, progressive evolution; we purge past 'bad' actions, often from previous lives, through suffering in the present. This can be more positive than it sounds; the belief is that you can set straight your own spiritual record and so find peace of mind in the process. Giftedness or innate wisdom are positive karmic attributes.

Another of the views Ken Wilber describes is the **psychological** one: that repressed emotions cause illness. This idea is integral to the holistic approach and the whole concept of body–mind. If we don't clear our emotional distress our bodies carry it in the form of 'dis–ease'. I hold strongly to this view because my experience tells me that my emotions are completely tied up with how I feel physically; an obvious example being a tension headache. It has been possible for me to discharge repressed emotion and change the way I feel and move in my body. However, there is the danger of 'over psychologising' physical symptoms. This can lead to guilt and more stress because a person can say to herself that if only she could 'sort out' her thinking or emotions then her physical symptoms would automatically disappear. This may not be so. And then to feel bad for remaining ill is disastrous.

Following this there is the **gnostic** view, in which illness is viewed as an illusion and we can only be free of it when we see that the material world in which we live is a dream, an illusion. Spirit is the only reality and spirit is free from illness. This is closely related to the **existential** view – that illness doesn't have meaning, it only has the meaning we choose to give it. There is also the **magical** view: that illness is retribution; you are suffering because you had a bad thought about somebody, or you mustn't be too happy because something bad is bound to happen. I often hear people say that they are being punished through their ill health. This is quite closely related to the fundamentalist Christian view.

The **Buddhist** view is that we cannot escape from illness in the manifest world; it is part of life. Only when we have become enlightened and transcended this physical world can we be free of illness. Pain and discomfort are experiences that remind us we are human, we are fallible.

Finally there is the **scientific** view, where illness is seen as having a specific cause or causes, some of which can be determined, others of which are simply due to chance and are completely random. So there is only chance or necessity, with illness having no deeper meaning. This is similar to the medical view.

For me there is some truth in each of these categories. In fact it can be said that the term **holistic** combines several of the categories that Ken Wilber describes, eg New Age, psychological, existential and Buddhist. What seems important to me is that we cannot separate illness, treatments and their results from what we believe.

What women share

As women we have a huge investment in our health and well-being. We may often be more preoccupied with this than men because we are constantly responding to the demands of our cycles and changes. Potentially this puts us in touch with nature and her rhythms. This also offers us a way of being closer to one another because of what we share. We know what it is like to regularly suffer physical discomfort and yet get on with life and manage external demands, whether these be from our jobs or our family commitments (or both). When women live together in small groups we start menstruating at the same time, which I find amazing. And, fascinatingly, we know that our cycles are related to the moon. The earth is described as Mother, the moon as female. We have a rich heritage in our femaleness that reaches into the depths of human experience; of our 'human-beingness'. As women we have the opportunity to support one another and share a great deal of subjective experience about our bodies.

In her book *What Makes Women Sick* Lesley Doyal says that 'despite their undoubted heterogeneity, women do have important things in common... All share broadly similar bodily experiences, even though the meanings they attach to them may vary dramatically... Bodies do impose very real (though varying) constraints on women's lives as well as offering enormous potential, and this is evidenced by the fact that the fight for bodily self-determination has been a central feature of feminist politics across very different cultures.'[3]

How women are taught to view their bodies

In *What Makes Women Sick* Lesley Doyal's focus is on the social origins of many of women's health problems, as well as our need for control over our own bodies. She describes the social construction of health and sickness and points out marked inequalities, both in quality of health for women from different racial backgrounds and classes and in access to conventional medical care. Such differences are bound to be evident within the availability of bodywork therapies, most especially because these are still predominantly confined to the private sector.

The medical profession itself is very much run along patriarchal lines with structures and hierarchies. This can lead to a disregard of the needs of individuals. For example, I think that the length of time on duty and resulting lack of sleep for junior hospital doctors seems to be a 'toughening-up' process verging on abuse. Describing her experience as a busy doctor, Christiane Northrup says 'As a good daughter of patriarchy, I worshipped at the altar of efficiency and productivity... Why did I feel so guilty whenever I rested?'[4]

Dr Northrup goes on to say 'our culture gives girls the message that their bodies, their lives and their femaleness demand an apology. Have you noticed how often women apologise?... If we must apologise for our very existence from the day we are born, we can assume that our society's medical system will deny us the wisdom of our "second-class" bodies. In essence, patriarchy blares out the message that women's bodies are inferior and must be controlled.'[5]

Do we internalise that something is basically wrong with our bodies? We feel we have to control natural odours that we deem to be essentially offensive. We may be either afraid of our natural processes, disgusted or embarrassed by them. You could say that our bodies have been 'medicalised' before we were born, our natural biological conditions often being viewed as medical conditions. Medicine itself is pathologically focused and often comes from a place of fear about what can go wrong. This can sometimes be self-fulfilling. Medical science mostly studies illness rather than health. I think it is a false belief that technology will save us and that it is possible to control and quantify everything. A result of this is that as individuals we ignore or do not trust our inner guidance systems and our own healing ability.

The difference between healing and cure

Caroline Myss says, 'Healing and curing are not the same thing. A "cure" occurs when one has successfully controlled or abated the physical progression of an illness. Curing a physical illness, however, does not necessarily mean that the emotional and psychological stresses that are a part of the illness are also alleviated. In this case it is highly possible, and often probable, that an illness will recur.'[6] Dr Sue Morrison, a holistic doctor working at the Marylebone Integrated Health Practice in London, suggests that as doctors 'we tend to cure a symptom rather than an illness.'

Healing is an active internal process and is to do with our own power. Curing is passive; we give the power to the doctor or alternative practitioner and expect an external treatment, and surgery or medication is used to eliminate or mask our symptoms. Unfortunately this external treatment doesn't necessarily address whatever contributed to the symptom in the first place. Lynne McTaggart states, 'Healing isn't simply a matter of finding the right drug or right operation, but a complex process of accepting responsibility for your own life.'[7]

The following story illustrates this difference, as well as the importance of healing ourselves on all levels of our being. (It also highlights how skilled and patient practitioners need to be when working with survivors of sexual and/or physical abuse.) Christine Steer writes:

'I am a disabled women of fifty-two, married with two grown-up children. I suffer with constant – and often severe – pain in my spine and limbs, with weakness and numbness in the limbs. I need to use a wheelchair outside of my home. My disability is due to brain-stem[8] damage caused by severe physical abuse in childhood. I also have some Arachnoiditis.[9]

Over the last thirty years I have had experience of many different bodywork therapies including: physiotherapy, osteopathy, reflexology, acupuncture, spiritual healing, aromatherapy massage/healing and osteopathy with cranial osteopathy. For the last eight years I have also been having psychotherapy, this being mainly focused on psychosynthesis and gestalt. I have spent a great deal of my time in psychotherapy focusing on my body, learning to like it and look after it, rather than hating and abusing it.

I have – until recently – been desperate to be "cured", and I've gone from one bodywork therapist to another in the hope of being cured. I've now reached a point where I can accept my disability and accept that a cure may never happen.

However, I *do* get considerable relief from my pain by having monthly treatments from an osteopath who has cranial expertise. Since seeing this osteopath my pain level has very gradually decreased to a level where, for most of the time, it is bearable and I can manage without painkillers during the day; although I do still need very strong painkillers at night.

Another very important part of my healing has been massage. I have had six years of fortnightly, then later monthly, sessions. At first I would not get undressed and was terrified of touch. Very gradually, as I began to trust, I was able to take my top clothes off and allow myself to be massaged, although only for a very limited time to begin with. During massage I was able to access my memories of the physical and sexual abuse I suffered as a child; these memories were stored in my body. Massage also helped to release a lot of my locked-in emotions. I was then able to work through these memories and emotions in my psychotherapy sessions. I no longer have any memories surfacing during massage. Massage is now a thoroughly enjoyable experience and eases a lot of the tension in my body and so helps to reduce my pain level. It also enables me to feel good about my body.

I have found that spiritual healing brings about very deep change on an emotional level and is able to heal very old and deep painful wounds.

I would just like to say that I believe that cranial osteopathy and aromatherapy massage, and even spiritual healing, would not have worked for me in isolation. They have worked well, for me, simply because I've experienced them in conjunction with my psychotherapy. This means that I have been working on all four aspects of myself – body, mind, emotions and spirit – *together* and not trying to treat each aspect as a separate entity.'

Death does not have to be a medical failure

I believe we need to put death and dying into a different – a holistic – light as well. Dying is part of our living. Death is not a failure. We can be supported into death and, if we are granted enough time, the weeks or months preceding our death can be a time of incredible healing, especially in our relationships. There is a point at which we need a 'death midwife', not a medical team using technology to keep us alive. This is not to undervalue the wonderful life-saving procedures that doctors and nurses do carry out, it is simply to say we need a different awareness.

The hospice movement is a wonderful bridge between life and death, where death is accepted and the quality of life enhanced as much as possible before death comes. Bodywork therapies are being used more extensively in hospices because of the comfort and contact they bring. Here the medical and the alternative/complementary are brought together. Healing and death are not mutually exclusive; we can be facing death in a more fully realised way. Consciously facing death invariably means living life much more fully and deeply.

Steven Levine, a poet and teacher of meditation, speaks of his work with the dying in one of his books, *Healing into Life and Death*: 'There were those with whom we sat on death-watch, whose dying expressed a wholeness of being; their hearts were so open, their spirits so fully released that it was evident how well they had become during the weeks and months of their dying. How much healing had occurred! They were more healed, more whole at the moment of their dying than at any time in their life. They had healed into death, their business finished, their future wide open.'[10]

My body, myself; taking responsibility

'Healing requires taking action. It is not a passive event,' says Caroline Myss. 'If you want to stay passive then medical care is the most appropriate form of treatment.'[11] Getting well can be an incredible journey that really does change people's lives.

Tragedies and illnesses obviously often happen outside our conscious control. We are then genuine victims. It is believed by many healers that when bad or difficult things happen we are unconsciously or on a spiritual or soul level choosing the experience to help us learn or grow in some way. In my experience I have found this idea easier to embrace in retrospect, with some distance in time between now and the actual experience. At the time it is the last thing I want to hear and I think those who try to point out the value in our suffering, unfortunately often in a self-righteous way, need to think twice. However, we can always learn from whatever happens to us. In the Chinese language the symbol for crisis and opportunity is the same. I may not choose to have a bad time but how I respond to it and what I am able to learn from it will affect how I grow and change as an individual. This does not mean that we should attempt to deny the terror, fear and anger at becoming seriously ill. It means finding ways of being with and coming through these painful times. It may also involve finding ways of coping with acute or chronic physical pain.

The power of thought and creative visualisation

How we think about ourselves and what we picture in our minds is crucial to our health. Positive or negative thinking has a direct chemical effect on the body. Every tissue and organ in our body is controlled by a complex interaction of hormones secreted by our endocrine glands and circulated in the blood stream. The pituitary gland, which is located in the middle of the head just below the brain, controls this. The output of these hormones from the pituitary is then controlled by chemical secretions and nerve impulses from the hypothalamus, the neighbouring part of the brain. Research is taking place about just how brain chemicals are related to emotions and thoughts.[12] Dr Bernie Segal states, 'We can change the body by dealing with how we feel. If we ignore our despair, the body receives a "die" message. If we deal with our pain and seek help, then the message is "Living is difficult but desirable", and the immune system works to keep us alive.'[13]

'Mind over matter' is a phrase often used in a simplistic, sometimes disparaging, way. Perhaps a better phrase is 'mind and matter'. The use of the power of the mind within complementary therapies is intrinsic to the philosophies underlying them. Often terms such as 'guided imagery' or 'creative visualisation' are used. Everything that has ever been created or accomplished was imagined first, created in thought form. Visualisation is the ability to create an idea or mental picture in your mind. Your images can be self-fulfilling prophecies and using this idea you can become what you visualise yourself to be.

Thought is creative and the theory is that there is no ultimate reality other than what thought creates. Creative energy is neither solid nor restricted and the physical world of form originates in something other than form itself. By aligning ourselves, or making a connection, and using our will we can tap into this force. 'There is absolutely no difference in the power that brings anything from the world of waves into the world of particles, and the power that brings your thoughts or mental pictures into form'[14] and '. . . think of manifesting as nothing more than transforming waves of possibilities into particles of reality.'[15]

When we are small we learn how to feel about ourselves and about life by the way the adults around us are doing so. If you lived with fearful, negative-thinking parents then you will have learned a lot of negative things about yourself and the world. This then affects your whole reality; you will expect the world to be unsafe and unsupportive. This is not to blame the parents. They could not have taught us what they didn't know.

This whole phenomenon is based on the idea that when you have a thought it goes out into the universe, into what seems like space around you. However, this is not simply space around you; it is a huge magnetic energy field that is full of activity, including sound and light waves, and millions of people's thoughts. These thoughts are not necessarily active all the time. Most thoughts simply fade out like a firework. They are short lived and in themselves quite insignificant. But more powerful, repetitive, emotionally charged thoughts actually have a much longer life and they become a strong vibration. They then gather together with other thoughts that are vibrating on a similar wavelength. Think of the positively charged atmosphere and energy in the room when you are talking with like-minded people; a meeting of minds with 'soul mates'.

The energy of thought itself is neutral. It is what we do with it that is either negative or positive. Deepak Chopra describes two qualities that are inherent in consciousness – attention and intention. 'Attention energizes, and intention transforms. Whatever you put your attention on will grow stronger in your life. Whatever you take your attention away from will wither, disintegrate and disappear.'[16]

Imagining an event before it happens actually puts neuromuscular processes to work. A single, positive image is stronger than many words; the brain thinks in pictures. We are likely to attract to us what we think about the most, believe in most strongly, expect on the deepest levels, and imagine most vividly. If you are anxious, negative, insecure or fearful you will not only tend to notice and then focus on the negative qualities of what happens for you, you will also tend to attract the very experiences, people or situations you are seeking to avoid. If you are positive, you will attract those things that confirm your positive expectations. The force of attraction is built into the magnetic and electrical nature of our planet. The energy that moves the planet also moves us.

In a creative visualisation session the person may be guided through a creative journey by a therapist. The therapist asks the client to close her eyes, bring her focus inside herself and respond either to the therapist's guiding story or to suggestions (see Chapter 9, HYPNOTHERAPY). Firstly, deep relaxation is very important to bring the brain into what is called the alpha brainwave level, a meditative state of mind. Creative visualisation involves using the right side of the brain to create the images and feelings. It then sends messages to the left side of the brain to work with it to create the change(s) desired.[17]

Creative visualisation is used as a therapeutic tool by therapists and healers. It is not a substitute for good listening, interacting or hands on/off healing. However it can be used as a method of self-direction; you can picture a desired outcome, or set goals, using images and affirmations. The primary benefits of creative visualisation are to bring about relaxation and peace of mind. It also helps with releasing limiting thoughts and emotions, raising self-esteem, establishing and attaining goals, clarifying questions and puzzles, healing relationships and encouraging physical healing. Really there are no limits. Here is my own story.

As a way of coping with the pain in my back, I began to meditate and visualise the pain. Once during meditation I felt I connected with everyone with back pain throughout the world, as if our pain at that moment was a collective energy. I wept and felt comforted. I didn't know that visualisation was a therapeutic tool; I had no idea. I drew the pain, talked to it and myself and definitely started to connect with the fact that who I was as a person, how I related to this experience and what I felt and thought were all tied up with my healing process. I also used visualisation to support me in my recovery from bulimia. Once I pictured myself slipping down stone steps that were covered in my own vomit. All of a sudden I saw several arms and hands reaching out to help lift me out of the vomit. They were the arms of friends. I knew from that moment that I had a choice, that others cared for me and that I could care more for myself. The forced rest, a result of the back injury, meant that I had time to really go into myself and take a long hard look.

Many of the therapies described in this book use visualisation techniques. For example, the chapter on CHI GUNG, which predates acupuncture, uses visualising the organs and chi pathways for healing. From chi gung came on the one side TAI CHI (strength and health), and on the other martial arts (using visualisation to throw an enemy off balance).

Both FELDENKRAIS (see Chapter 10) and KINESIOLOGY (see Chapter 7) use very subtle movements that include the use of visualisation to drastically change the body's abilities and responses.

Within humanistic psychotherapy GESTALT uses visualisation to work with inner bodily sensation, giving form to and options for new emotional choices. HYPNOSIS uses the power of the imagination and pre-dates the modern humanistic and transpersonal psychotherapies by a long way.

In the 1770s Franz Anton Mesmer used hypnosis with his magnetic healing techniques. In the twentieth century Freud labelled the unconscious mind and gave the concept of imagination a much more scientific status. Jung, a student of Freud, took the idea of the unconscious mind and created the term 'collective unconscious', opening up Freud's more medical model into spiritual and archetypal realms of thought, such as the gateway to the unconscious mind. The imagination became a modern way to spiritual guidance and self-discovery.

There are also psycho-educational therapies such as neuro-linguistic programming (NLP). Along with auditory and kinesthetic senses, NLP uses visually constructed and visually remembered images to 'reframe' experiences that may have been traumatic (see Appendix II).

In HEALING spiritual healers often combine visualisation with hands-on energy work. This may be through encouraging the client to work with an image that has come to her mind spontaneously, or it may be through the use of psychic imagery that the healer experiences in his or her own mind or has been given by an internal or external source (this will depend on the healer's belief system). In DISTANT HEALING the healer uses deliberately formed images or psychic information in the form of pictures to extend/channel healing at a distance.

Some forms of meditation use focusing on an image to calm the mind. This is very different to creative visualisation as an action, as most meditation is more about emptying the mind and detaching from images and thoughts rather than working with them.

Emille Coué wrote *Self Mastery Through Conscious Auto-suggestion* (1922) and *How to Practise Suggestion and Autosuggestion* (1923), introducing POSITIVE AFFIRMING as a technique that can be used by itself or be included in a visualisation exercise. Positive affirmations counteract previous negative decisions we have made, or negative messages we have been given and have continued to give ourselves. They are a form of positive thinking and are much more powerful when imagery is added. Coué's famous affirmation is 'Every day, in every way, I am getting better and better.'

Self-help

Positive affirmations: firstly, you need to create a positive affirmation. This needs to be a short, to-the-point statement, written in the present tense, beginning with an 'I', and including your own name. You are going to write it out several times so the shorter the better. For example, 'I, Delcia, have radiant health.' Affirmations are about achieving goals. Goals can be material, such as earning more money or having the holiday of your dreams, or can be about a quality that you would like to have, such as being more accepting of yourself, or they can be about relationships or having a baby. The possibilities are endless. The words need to be exactly right for you. By putting them in the present tense you have a felt experience of what it would really be like to actually have this thing or quality, even though for the moment you haven't actually got it and you may have strong doubts that you could ever really have it.

Next take a piece of paper, make two columns and write down your affirmation in full at the top of the left-hand column. It is likely that immediately after this you will have a negative thought. A doubt may have popped into your mind. Write this thought down straight away at the top of the right-hand column. Then you return to the left-hand column and write out your positive statement again. Up will come the same or another negative thought. Again, write this down in the right-hand column. Repeat this process backwards and forwards for a minimum of twelve times. You should find that gradually the negative response weakens. If this doesn't happen and you get stuck, this means that your positive affirmation is too big a leap for you and you need to rewrite it, changing it slightly, to make it more of a possibility. Or there may be some other doubt or negative belief that needs to be dealt with before you can work on your original positive affirmation. However, as the negative thoughts diminish you start to believe in your positive affirmation. You start to feel what it is like to be or have this quality or goal. In my own example, I picture myself in radiant health: full of energy, bright eyes, clear skin, happy, bouncing along, walking, swimming or dancing.

The above is one way of working with positive affirmations. There are many others such as writing your statement on a piece of paper and sticking it in a place you look at regularly, like on your mirror or fridge door. You can make a tape of affirmations and listen to them regularly; you can sing them, or get someone to say them back to you.

As well as Emile Coué, other New Age writers and therapists who have had a major influence in the whole area of positive affirmations and creative visualisation include therapists and writers such as Shakti Gawain, Dina Glauberman, Bernie Siegel and Gill Edwards (see Selected Reading). There are many more individuals and systems, using the power of the imagination and the mind (eg see The Silva Mind Method mentioned in Appendix II). It is important to remember that everything that is created starts with a vision, a thought or a voice. The scientist who discovered DNA saw a spiral staircase. Scientists have hunches, dreams and visions. They then work hard to develop theories and evidence to bring the original image into the material world.

A word of warning: imagination without subsequent action/behaviour change remains pure fantasy. To use visualisation successfully to help with physical symptoms or emotional pain you must be willing to act on what you learn from your own mind.

Self-help

Creative visualisation: although it is potentially very beneficial to do visualisations with the help of a therapist, since our imaginations are always available to us this area of bodywork is the most accessible for self-help. You can use pre-recorded tapes (see Resources) or allow your own mind to take you on a journey, seeing what images come to you and giving yourself time to see if you can give them meaning or interpret them. Here are some practical guidelines for self-help:

People visualise in different ways. You may need to sit or lie down comfortably and close your eyes. You may experience any of the following, in any combination:

- clear and specific pictures
- symbolic forms
- words heard
- sounds
- non-specific sense of something or an intuitive knowing.

Don't judge what happens for you and take these often subtle signs through your senses seriously. To explore them you can draw them, describe them aloud, or allow yourself to follow your thoughts, noticing what images or words come to you as the process unfolds.

A controlled environment is essential. Apart from physical comfort, this may include dim lighting, no interruptions, limited outside noises and access to music and/or a tape recorder – (the session can then be reused in the future). You need an adequate amount of time put aside; it is important not to rush. It is useful to have identified a specific need (eg you have a pain somewhere that you want to alleviate) as you need to feel that you are in control.

For reaching goals choose something that is realistic to achieve. Put yourself into your pictures. Make sure you complete the exercise. Make your pictures look as if you already have what you want. In the case of a pain somewhere, for example, imagine that part of your body healthy and pain-free. In my example about positive affirming, I added seeing myself full of energy and bouncing along. So put strong emotion into the pictures and emphasise your senses. If your thoughts drift, don't judge yourself, just go back to the subject. Repeat your visualisation throughout the day. This involves a commitment to exploring, discovering and changing what are sometimes your deepest and most basic attitudes towards life. The creative abilities of the mind need to be fine-tuned; this takes practice, like playing an instrument. You need to be gentle with yourself and allow this to happen.

Chapter Three
Touch and Contact

'. . . for each of us our response to touch is rooted in the early experience of touch in our lives and therefore involves all levels of our being. Our attitude to touch inevitably taps into primitive and fundamental aspects of who we each are as individuals' (Bernd Eiden).[1]

Most of the therapies described involve touch of one kind or another. Exceptions are acupuncture, which involves needles, the psychotherapies and energy movement systems. These latter categories may still involve touch. For example, the acupuncturist touches when she takes the pulses, and the psychotherapist or movement therapist may touch to make contact at a certain point in the session, or may hold the person whilst they express grief, pain and so on. The rest of the therapies require the person to sit or lie down, for all or most of the session, and receive touch contact from the therapist, either directly on the skin or through the clothes.

If you are recovering from addiction, ie an eating disorder, alcohol or drugs, then bodywork can support you through this. The nurturing therapies, such as holistic massage, are particularly good because they offer you an experience of receiving a caring, respectful touch that is accepting of you. An addiction invariably masks a person's bad feelings about him or herself and this behaviour is a way of moving away from this discomfort. Having your body stroked, held and gently worked on can give you an experience of respect that at the time you are unable to give to yourself. This helps you to build self-esteem.

Touch and the use of language

We regularly use metaphors to illustrate the body-mind connection, such as 'put your back into it'. Here are some specific ones about touch: we talk about rubbing people up the wrong way, we grapple with problems, we have abrasive or prickly personalities. We talk about the personal touch, getting in touch or in contact, the magic touch, a soft touch. Some of us are thick-skinned, others thin-skinned, we can be touchy or tetchy. Some people get under our skin. We can get out of touch or lose our grip. We may feel snug or cling to another. An unfeeling person may be described as callous which is derived from the Latin, *callus*, meaning hard skin. We need to hold on to someone or something, get a firm grip, or grasp the point. A good movie or story is gripping. To make sure we have got the reality of an idea we put our finger on it.

The use of language generally supports our view of ourselves as having a body and mind that are not separate. We often bring together thought, emotion and our own anatomy. Someone is a pain in the neck or spineless; we refer to gut feelings as our instincts, our intuitions; we may be told to 'put your back into it' – that is make more effort. We have broken hearts; we get things off our chests; we handle things; keep others at arm's length; get hopping mad and so on. All these metaphors are referring to what is termed the body-mind. There is no such thing as psychosomatic, meaning 'it's all in the mind'. Everything is psychosomatic. 'Psycho' refers to the mind, and somatic to the body. Even accidents are more likely to happen when we have a lot on our mind, or feel generally stressed, and this power can be used positively, as discussed in the previous chapter.

Touch itself can raise all kinds of issues, especially for women who have been abused. There is also the issue of absence of touch, such as when a mother has postnatal depression, or when four-hourly feeds were the norm and mothers were taught to let the baby cry and not pick it up. Whatever the issue, trust is a key factor.

Your skin

Massage practitioner Kate Williams says: 'I believe that the experience of the world through our skin is an important part of the process through which we inform ourselves about what is happening in our lives and how we organise ourselves internally in response.'[2] The skin is a highly sensitive, tactile organ and is the largest organ of the body. It receives the signals that come to us from our environment and then relays them to our brain, where they can be deciphered. This is a two-way process. Another function is that it also picks up signals from our inner world. As far as we know it is the earliest sensory system functioning in all living creatures. It is the first sense through which we communicate and is a crucial part of our nervous system. Our skin is our emotional mirror. It tingles with excitement and goes numb with shock, we turn red when we are embarrassed and blanch when afraid. Our physical health can be assessed through our skin's colour, dryness, moistness, and texture.

Skin has a multitude of physical functions. For instance, it protects us from toxic materials or organisms and bacteria in our environment; its surface area has millions of sensory receptors receiving the stimuli of heat, cold, pressure, pain and, of course, touch; it breathes, metabolises and stores fat, produces keratin (the protein that forms the basis of our nails and hair); it regulates our temperature, and makes us water-proof and dust-proof. When we are touched, in whatever form, the nerve cells on the skin receiving the stimulus activate generators of weak electrical currents. Our skin is like an external part of our nervous system and so a lot of electrical activity occurs when we are touched.

The emotional and physical significance of touch

The actual lack of touch when we are small is experienced as a separation anxiety: a lack of contact, of connection, of feeling contained. This is the same as when a lover leaves us. Our bodies can literally ache from the loss of physical contact. People who live alone, and especially elderly people, may not be touched from one week to the next. Whatever the reasons for this lack of contact, the body and therefore the person experiences loneliness.

How we are touched from the beginning of our lives affects our growth and development. Ashley Montague writes: 'Where touching begins, there love and humanity also begin – within the first minutes following birth.' He also states '... it would greatly help towards our rehumanization if we would pay closer attention to the need we all have for tactile experience.' Even more startling, if babies are not touched through caressing, handling, carrying and cuddling they can die from a disease called marasmus, from the Greek meaning wasting away. 'Extreme sensory deprivation in other respects, such as light and sound, can be survived, as long as the sensory experiences at the skin are maintained.'[3] This is how important caring touch is. The present rise in books and courses about baby massage is an encouraging development (see Chapter 5). Indeed, since touch has been proved to be essential to the growing infant, it follows that it must be important throughout life.

The very need for infant massage reflects the inhibition that many Westerners have around touch. There are far-reaching consequences. For instance, according to a study by Dr Mary Ainsworth on rearing practices among the Ganda of East Africa, the majority of mothers carry their infant on their backs and the babies spend most of their waking hours being held by someone. Mothers constantly gently pat or stroke their baby. The consequence of this is that the rate of sensorimotor development is accelerated in most babies. They sit, stand, crawl and walk much earlier than the average baby in Western societies.[4]

These Ugandan women, with their infants on their backs, know when the child needs to urinate, defecate or feed. A further study of the Netsiliks on the Boothia Peninsula in the Canadian Arctic of the Northwest Territories by Richard James de Boer in 1967 shows that the infants' needs are anticipated by the mother tactually; they communicate with each other through their skin. The infant is placed inside its mother's fur parka on her back and is held comfortably and securely by a sash formed into a sling. 'The infant wears tiny diapers fashioned from caribou skins, but otherwise it snuggles naked against its mother's skin.' The front of the baby is in direct contact with its mother and its back is completely encased in fur to protect it from the arctic weather.[5] Another researcher of the Netsiliks, Dr Otto Schaeffer, found that when he asked a mother how she knew when her baby needed to urinate, she was astonished by such a question; any capable mother knew by the movement of her baby's legs. This particular culture is described as being based on mutually altruistic interpersonal relationships. Dominance–subservience relationships are absent in parental relationships and there is a harmonic balance between the Netsilik individual and her society.[6] The same kind of contact is found in the Arapesh society, New Guinea. Where tactile experience is high between adult and child and is sensitive and enjoyed by both, it can be generally said that aggression in adults and children is low.[7]

Obviously touch is influenced a great deal by culture, but every family is different and everyone has their own level of comfort in terms of how and when they want to be touched, and how much physical space they need around them. I believe these needs should be respected and it is important for us as adults to let others know what is right for us.

Generally speaking in the UK, women are more likely to reach out and touch than men. This can be attributed to internalised preparation, from early in life, for girls to be mothers/nurturers and boys to be providers on a materialistic level. Touch between genders can often be sexualised and therefore limited; it becomes a danger zone and there can be confusion between general intimacy and having sex.

Touch and therapy

Since our experience of touch and our associations with it are strongly influenced by our early experiences – including pre-verbal ones – how a bodywork therapist touches us can be a very powerful experience. It can release profound emotion and needs to be used with care and appropriate backup for the client. The therapist needs her own support and supervision to manage this well.

Unfortunately in our culture, where touch is so often associated exclusively with sexual gratification, therapists must have great integrity and never use their clients to meet their own needs for contact or for sexual gratification. The absolute exclusion of any sexual touch must be guaranteed.

Touch and physical and sexual abuse

If you have been physically or sexually abused then clearly your experience of touch has been damaging for you. It has been invasive, probably painful and disrespectful. The touch you received was to do with the needs of the person giving it, your needs were disregarded and you were not listened to. This kind of touch violation understandably can lead to difficulties in feeling comfortable with touch and intimacy later in life. Trust is a key issue.

During a bodywork session you may experience felt and visual flashbacks to the abuse situation, which prevent you feeling what is happening in the moment. I have worked with massage and healing survivors of abuse who have experienced my hands as the hands of their abuser, even though they know that they are being touched by me and that I am a safe person to be touched by. One client said 'I know it's you and I knows it's your hand, but I feel my father's hand.' When caught up in a memory you may find it difficult or impossible to tell your practitioner because you are experiencing the same feelings of powerlessness as you did when you were being abused. Working with the right therapist is essential and this is discussed in the next chapter.

Geraldine is in her fifties, and soon to be a grandmother for the first time. She is a survivor of both physical and sexual abuse:

'I once had experience of a massage practitioner who really hurt me because she pressed down far too hard on my body and never once asked me whether she was hurting me or what kind of touch I needed, whereas the practitioner I see now always asks me several times during a massage about whether the kind of touch she is giving is OK.'

For all clients, the therapist carries a great deal of responsibility for when and how she touches and she needs to have access to a subtle and highly differentiated sense of touch in herself. In our culture such an ability is quite rare and therapists of different bodywork disciplines learn and develop this through training and experience. The experience of receiving appropriate touch in a therapeutic setting from a skilled therapist is, I believe, one of the most significant experiences any human being can have. In this way your whole being is recognised and honoured.

Chapter Four

Finding a Practitioner or Therapist

You may well be thinking 'how on earth do I choose the therapy and therapist best for me?' This is a genuine problem and there is no easy answer. The majority of the treatments work for all sorts of conditions and people often use more than one therapy concurrently. It is important, however, not to have too many bodywork therapies at once. It is much better to have a series of sessions with one practitioner and see how that benefits you. You may then go on to try something else if you wish. I am wary of events such as alternative health and mind, body, spirit exhibitions where there are many therapies on offer that people can try. I think this should be discouraged. Although most therapies are very gentle and subtle, they are powerful and, although I do not think any major harm can come from trying out more than one at once, I do know from my own experience that the body can simply become overwhelmed with input and you can feel confused and disoriented. Having said this, often when people are using more than one therapy they are having a bodywork therapy together with an alternative medicine such as homoeopathy or herbalism and this can work very well. For instance, for me a good mix is cranial osteopathy, massage, subtle energy healing and homoeopathy. I like to have at least one session in one of the hands–on therapies a month and then have homoeopathy when I need it.

Generally speaking gathering information and developing discernment is part of our learning as we take greater responsibility for our health. It can demand being able to look at different beliefs and approaches with an open mind and from there make decisions based on sound information. This still involves taking a risk – the risk to do something different.

A lot of fear from trying something different can come about as a result of other people's concerns and scepticism, or simply their ignorance. As I mentioned earlier, I was still in considerable pain following nine months of osteopathic treatment after my back injury. A relative very kindly suggested that as it really wasn't helping me I should stop it. I knew deep inside, however, that it was helping me, but that it was just taking time. I simply had to trust my gut instinct and hope for the best. I'm glad that I did.

Another aspect of discernment involves getting clear about what you are seeking and learning how to judge the quality of who and what you are drawn to. The therapies in this book vary in how unsafe they are in inexperienced hands. For example, an inappropriate osteopathic adjustment can seriously hurt you; needling the wrong acupuncture points can make things worse. Although many of these therapies are gentle – and some definitely are not – they have powerful effects. You need to make sure that your practitioner is trained properly in the therapy she is offering. You may want to find out what the training requirements are (see Resources). Some therapies can be learned quickly, especially the metaphysical ones. Often practitioners have natural, inborn healing gifts, which they then develop further. Care needs to be taken that your practitioner has a mature attitude and can relate to you appropriately, as well as be skilled at what she does. Angie, a physiotherapist, psychotherapist and healer herself, refers to this in the account she sent me:

'There are many new therapies attracting numerous people to train. Unfortunately this is a "get rich quick", "get on the bandwagon" time. I believe a practitioner is formed from many life experiences, which enrich us if we have used those opportunities to work on ourselves, and to resolve inner and outer conflicts. A couple of weekend courses will never form a true practitioner of the integrity and experience that I believe is necessary to be able to "hold" the client as they become more aware of themselves and disorganise in order to change.'

Professional support and supervision

I believe that proper support is essential to good practice. Professional supervision is an integral part of psychotherapeutic and counselling work. However, its value is less known about and appreciated within more general bodywork therapy. Supervision does not mean having someone checking up on you; it means having someone or several people to help you understand problems that inevitably arise when working with clients. Each of us have blind spots; we simply do not see all there is to see in a given situation. I personally regard supervision as an essential component of post-qualifying practice and not simply for trainees. It provides a confidential forum for support, and for getting clear around issues that arise when working with clients. Ethics and codes of practice, and individual case management, as well as managing client-therapist relationship issues and generally building and managing a practice, are some of the issues therapists bring to supervision. When therapists take their own needs seriously they are able to maintain their effectiveness with their clients.

I believe it is important that therapists inform their clients about how they as therapists receive support for themselves, and to reassure them of the strict confidentiality that surrounds this.

Finding information

Part 2 of this book gives you an introduction to the most widely known bodywork therapies and how they can help you. Therapists will vary depending on where you live. If you live in London or a big city there will be a wide choice available to you locally. If you live in a rural area, there may be less choice, but there is still likely to be some. This still leaves the question of which is the best *available* therapy for you.

Word of mouth is often the best way. Good treatments stand on their own merit. Knowing that others, whose judgment you trust, have been helped has to be more reliable than advertisements, books and the like. Also, by being open and talking with other women about particular symptoms, it is amazing to discover how many people suffer from similar problems and how much information can be shared, as well as support given.

However, information can, of course, be gained from other sources and, if you don't know anyone who has tried a particularly therapy, or indeed any complementary or alternative therapy, then reading about it is helpful. You can borrow **books** from the library, buy books if and when you can afford them, and educate yourself about your problem and the alternatives available. If you have a medical diagnosis you can educate yourself about the anatomical and pathological nature of your condition. You can visit specialised bookshops and put yourself on the mailing lists of holistic health and therapy and personal growth publishers (see Resources).

Contact the national organisation representing the therapy you are interested in. These professional bodies keep lists of qualified, registered members. Many of these are listed in Resources. If the specific therapy organisation is not available, refer to a more general CAM body, which should have information about all the therapies available.

You can also join or receive information from **self-help organisations** and groups for particular conditions. Such organisations are likely to have begun from a conventional medicine point of view, so may have only limited information on what alternatives are available, but they do try to provide a broad-based approach for members, so they may be worth a try.

You can pick up **leaflets** written by local practitioners in **health-food shops, natural health centres, libraries and wholefood cafés**.

Exhibitions are generally good places to educate yourself and try out a therapy that appeals. Only one therapy at a time is advisable. Often there are special offers on treatments or products. There are also always plenty of books to browse through at these events.

Local **natural health centres** often have open days or open evenings where you can go along and have a 'taster' session and talk to practitioners. Some **GPs** or **nurse practitioners, district nurses, health visitors, physiotherapists, occupational therapists** and so on are interested and knowledgeable, and could direct you.

If you have access to the **Internet** you can look up anything. I was moved to tears when I looked up night-terrors and read the stories of others who were just as confused and uncertain about the causes of this condition as I was. If you are suffering from something you can almost guarantee that someone else out there is suffering, too. You can also get in touch with a multitude of women's health organisations on the net. If you don't have personal access, use public Internet resources such as your library. Many towns now have Internet cafés.

If you are disabled

In my experience disability awareness in training courses for alternative and complementary therapists is minimal. Most practitioners who choose to specialise in working with disabled adults or children, or who meet this in their general day-to-day practice, learn about particular issues when they need to. As with society at large, I believe there is considerable room for improvement in awareness.

As a disabled person there are limitations and discomforts that you have had to learn to live with and that you take for granted; you may have had them all your life. An able-bodied practitioner is living in a different reality and so may have no idea at all about what life is really like for you. This means that two-way communication between you and your practitioner is even more important than for able-bodied clients.

An exciting new development within a charity called The Disability Foundation (see Resources) is the provision of a holistic approach to both conventional and complementary treatments and therapies offered to disabled people and their families. All the practitioners are disabled in some way themselves.

As a disabled person certain therapies may be not be appropriate for your particular condition. It is essential to discuss this with the practitioner concerned, who will take a medical history and check out any contraindications. You may want to consider taking along a support person or carer so that you can be clear about the kind of contract you are entering in receiving treatments or sessions with a practitioner. Find out whether the practitioner has successfully treated others with your condition in the past.

It is important that you feel able to inform your practitioner about your particular needs. If you experience difficulties in accepting your body's limitations, complex and difficult feelings may arise when you are touched in a respectful and caring way. You need a practitioner who feels comfortable about disability and who can accept your feelings without trying to 'fix' you.

Access to practitioners and therapists is obviously crucial if you have mobility problems of any kind. Some practitioners, especially spiritual healers and massage practitioners, do home visits. Like all home visiting, this may cost more because of travelling costs and time.

Most therapies can be adapted to meet the needs of different kinds of impairment. For instance, it is very possible that if you are not able to get up on to a treatment couch, your practitioner needs to be flexible and able to adapt her treatment to work with you seated or lying on the floor or a low bed. Safety is very important; you don't want to feel you have to get into any position that may mean you could fall or hurt yourself. Equally important is comfort.

If you are blind you will be unable to see the environment in which you are being treated; you will not be able to read the facial expressions of your practitioner or, if appropriate to the therapy, see where the treatment couch is. Your practitioner needs to be sensitive to your special needs. If you are profoundly deaf and you are receiving a treatment face down on the couch you will not be able to lip-read or sign to the practitioner. You will need to work out some form of communication with her before getting on to the couch, such as right arm up for 'It is okay' and left arm up for 'It is not okay' or 'please stop'.

If you are recovering from a stroke or have any condition that numbs or alters your sensations your practitioner needs to know. Be particularly careful around loss of sensation, as a practitioner could accidentally bruise or hurt you and you would not know because you could not feel it. Alternatively you may have heightened sensation.

Communication is so important. Make sure that your practitioner knows if there are any parts of your body you do not want touched. It is good to give as much information as possible about your disability but think about how much information you are prepared to give. For instance, does your disability mean that you may have any unusual physical responses, such as fits, or spasms, or coming out in a rash?

Expectations are also important. Be honest with yourself and your practitioner about them; are you hoping for a miracle cure? You can fall into this trap and then feel bitterly disappointed. It is good to value every bit of progress, no matter how small it may seem.

Complementary therapies may be available to you via your GP, or a charity. The kind of support and encouragement that can come from receiving touch that is therapeutic cannot be underestimated.

Coral McKenzie had a stroke in 1988 when she was just twenty-one years old. She was left with paralysis of her left arm and leg. She attends a day centre for disabled people in East London, where she receives regular massage treatments.

'I was told by the physiotherapists that they had done as much as they could do for me, and that now, because of the damage in my nervous system and because it had been so long since the stroke, nothing was going to change. I was not feeling positive or assertive, but since having massage I've taken on a different approach. I wasn't walking and now I'm even able to go down the road and cross it. My massage practitioner helped me overcome my fear of open spaces. I have put the breathing and relaxing into action. I can move my arm a lot better; before I could only lift it a little and that with great difficulty. It was so stiff. Now all the stiffness has gone.'

Self-help

Obviously self-help exercises will depend on the nature and severity of your disability. Move your limbs as much as possible. Very small, gentle movements are extremely beneficial, often more so than bigger movements. It is important to focus on what you can do, rather than what you can't. Self-massage in the form of rubbing your hands and shoulders can help you release tension and feel lighter.

If you have been sexually and/or physically abused

Many women are trying to recover from sexual and/or physical abuse. You will need a therapist who is aware of the kinds of problems you face. A bodywork therapist who has done some counselling training would be best, and/or a therapist who has worked on recovering from abuse herself. Your tolerance of any kind of insensitivity on the part of the therapist is likely to be extremely low, if not nil. Your tolerance of mistakes can be less than zero. Unfortunately this can stop you going to any other practitioner. I hope that the information here will prevent this.

You may well feel unwilling or unable to talk about your abuse. You could ask to talk for fifteen minutes or so to the practitioner before deciding whether or not to make a session time with her. If you meet before you commit, you don't have to give all the details. A good practitioner will recognise how ready you are or not to speak about your abuse experience(s). If the practitioner is insensitive or tries to press you when you are not ready, then go to someone else.

A bodywork therapist who works with female survivors of sexual abuse and who is a survivor herself suggests that bodywork therapies such as applied KINESIOLOGY can be preferable because the receiver's own body is telling her and the therapist what she needs. It is an active therapy in which she participates. This is very different from expecting yourself to lie passively and receive, for example, a massage. This can be too evocative of the original abuse situation. She writes:

'If you do want massage you need to seek a practitioner who

can adapt to your needs: perhaps to work through clothing, to be very patient in allowing the trust to build slowly between you. You may prefer receiving a massage to your head, neck and shoulders, remaining seated and clothed. You may find that what you would like in terms of touch and what you can actually handle at any one time are quite different things.'

There is evidence that the effects of sexual abuse are lessened by massage therapy. Research done at the Touch Research Institute, University of Miami School of Medicine concludes that, following a thirty-minute massage twice a week for one month, women reported being less depressed and less anxious, and their saliva cortisol (stress hormones) levels decreased.[1]

Susan came to one of my massage for women classes some years back. She writes:

'As I started learning massage I realised I had a real resilience to being touched, that in many ways it actually hurt me, although the pain was never really physical. I learned about how child abuse had affected me whenever anyone touched me, and that even taking my clothes off just in front of other women was extremely difficult.'

And another survivor of sexual abuse writes:

'I have received treatments that felt invasive and disrespectful of my body's wounds. Postural integration and standard physiotherapy were the worst. There seemed to be no account taken of my subjective experience, no awareness of "body armouring", of the emotional pain held in the body – or safe facilitation when releasing it. It was again as if someone was doing something to my body that hurt, yet I was being told it was "for my own good".'

When you have found a way to feel more connected to your body, you are likely to face dealing with memories that are stored in your muscles. Bodywork can really help you connect with these memories. Some people find that, once having started to feel the emotional pain held in their bodies, they then have counselling or psychotherapy. Excellent work is taking place where a bodywork therapist – often a massage practitioner or healer – is working alongside a counsellor or psychotherapist. The latter becomes the place in which the person can work through what has come up in the bodywork session. Some therapies combine massage and psychotherapy (see Chapter 9, BIODYNAMIC MASSAGE).

Good communication is the key issue here. You need to feel that your practitioner is really listening to you. Here is a quote from one of my massage and healing clients, who several years ago didn't want to be touched at all by anyone:

'One of the greatest benefits I got out of our work together was that I learned to have control over who I allowed to touch my body and how they touched it, because I was listened to by you. Being listened to is what stopped it from being abusive touch. I would like everyone that has a difficulty with their body, whether it's a disability or a problem with touch, to have some form of bodywork therapy because it teaches you to have a better relationship with your body.'

Fees

Your financial needs as a client
If you have a chronic condition – endometriosis, back pain, recurring cystisis or thrush and so on – you may be concerned about how much your treatments are going to cost over time. It is important to recognise that chronic conditions take time

to heal. There is a theory that for every year you have had the condition it takes one month of treatment. In my experience this seems quite accurate. Within holistic medicine you are not simply suppressing a symptom, you are changing the 'ground' in which the symptom is born; you are changing your body-mind.

I like to budget for my treatments. They are now built into my life as part of the resources I need, such as electricity, rent, car and so on. This means that I have this financial need in my consciousness and when I am considering what I need to earn this is included. New Age theories about abundance and prosperity are rather different from the political and feminist views of women as victims of an unjust economic system. When viewing the distribution and direct ownership of wealth in the world, it is absolutely true that women's oppression has a large economic component. Within many employment sections of our society we still have a way to go to reach equality with men.

I have found that the idea of 'prosperity consciousness' and the use of affirmations and visualisations has helped me transcend some of the gender influences when it comes to earning income. 'Prosperity consciousness' means that you are coming from a place of believing that you deserve and can create the level of wealth that you want in your life. Wealth here does not simply refer to sums of money or property, it means having a wealth of well-being as well as health and happiness. To prosper means to flourish, to succeed and to thrive. It is also based on the belief that there is enough for everybody and that if we give and receive openly and lovingly we can all do well. It is not based on a belief in scarcity; that we have to have winners and losers in society and that there is not enough to go round. The latter is called 'poverty consciousness'.

There is a lot of contention around payment for medical care. There is a view that when people pay for their treatments they have a higher level of commitment to personal responsibility than those who receive it for free. The professional relationship is more equal, not being based on welfare and dependency. On the other hand thousands of women, most especially single mothers and elderly women, who could benefit by receiving bodywork treatments genuinely cannot afford them. One of the contributors to this book said she found her chiropractic treatment for back pain quite successful but left before she should have because of the expense.

Another problem is that the NHS in the UK is very overstretched. Because of the success of modern technology and surgery, the public's expectations have increased. We are expecting to live longer with a better quality of health. For instance, hip replacements are now commonplace, as is open-heart surgery. But these are very expensive procedures and how they are paid for is a big question. I do believe, however, that much surgery could be avoided if more people had access to CAM earlier on in the development of their symptoms; CAM is also intrinsically a preventive medicine.

Here are some other comments from women:

'In general, I think due to the fees of alternative therapies they are not available to all women. Several of the therapies that I would like to try are too expensive. I would very much like to see therapies on offer at the GP's surgery, and although this is happening in some areas people usually have to pay.'

Catherine is in her early fifties and has been using a wide range of alternative and complementary therapies for over twenty years. She writes:

'I do have some concerns about the availability of different therapies and particularly the cost. However, I think that this is a difficult issue as I am not convinced that having complementary therapies available in the same way as allopathic medicine is necessarily the answer...I feel that the relationship between the therapist and client is a vital aspect of the healing and that the time given in sessions is important, so I would not want to see this diminished to the few minutes of a GP consultation. It is also necessary, in my opinion, to maintain the holistic approach of many of these therapies. However, I would also like to be able to have more freedom of choice in treatments available to me that are funded by my contributions to National Insurance.'

Here are some ideas about what you can do if you can't afford treatments or sessions:

- Go to a training school that runs a supervised clinic for its final year students. You can receive low-cost treatments and, because they are supervised, you get the benefit of the knowledge of experience.
- Go to a student who is coming towards the end of their training. All students of complementary therapies have to do individual case studies and need people to practise on. Check them out and if you feel good about their skills and their approach then you can get free treatment.
- If you have health insurance, some policies cover complementary therapies for a limited period of time.
- Many spiritual healers work on a donation basis. These healers are not usually doing healing for their living, or it may be their paid work but they are doing some voluntary work as well. These 'healing clinics' tend to be run by a group of healers who hire community premises or church halls for a few hours a week. You often do not get privacy in these situations but you can receive the benefits of laying-on-hand healing. The largest healing organisation providing

this service is the NFSH (see Resources).

- Most practitioners I know have concessionary fees; that is, they either have a sliding scale, offer low-cost sessions, or will negotiate with you.
- You could perhaps use the LETS scheme if there is one available in your area, or start a scheme.[2]
- You could talk to your GP and ask her or him if there is any way you could have access to complementary therapy, eg massage practitioner, aromatherapist, healer, counsellor. In some GP practices the fee is shared between the practice and the patient.
- If you are under medical care with a hospital, or if you know health visitors, community nurses, other medical personnel, ask them if they could put forward a request for provision of some of these therapies.
- You can experience many of these therapies by learning about them yourself, eg at adult education institutes or private classes. In this way you can empower yourself.
- You could create a self-help group, share information and experiences and find out together; you could invite a qualified practitioner to come and talk to you and share the cost.

The financial needs of the practitioner

The general public has little information about the challenges and costs of setting up and maintaining practice as a complementary practitioner. I want to mention them here so that you can have a more realistic view of what is involved.

Unfortunately, as yet there is little or no public funding for training courses. Over and over again I have met a strong vocational commitment amongst a large number of practitioners, a huge proportion of which are women. At the same time shortage of funds limits many of them. A conscientious therapist also needs to continue to have post-graduate training, professional supervision and attend to her own ongoing personal development or therapy while she is working with the public. As these therapies are not usually part of a public service the practitioners pay for all their own overheads, as well as marketing and advertising their own services.

Managing a business involves very different skills from practising the therapy itself. As these therapies aren't in the mainstream it can also mean the therapist has to overcome self-esteem issues before entering into a business wholeheartedly. I am hopeful that in years to come more and more opportunities will become available in the public sector for CAM therapists to be employed in primary health care, and so not need to be solely self-employed. However, the pioneering aspect of our work means that we need to sell ourselves to the public, the medical profession and the media in order to be taken seriously. This is a great challenge, especially for women who can find it hard to define and value themselves. As a result, female practitioners often charge less than their male colleagues, but this does not necessarily reflect their skills in any way.

Questions to ask a potential practitioner

Since word of mouth is likely to be the best way to get to know who may be good for you, make sure you are thorough about researching the practitioner's reputation.

When you speak with the practitioner – usually initially on the phone – see how you feel about what they say and how they say it. Do you like the sound of them? Do they answer your questions with ease and openness? Do you feel comfortable speaking with them? Do they seem to have clear boundaries concerning the way they work, such as length of sessions, fees, cancellation times, confidentiality and so on?

Look for a practitioner who you can talk with and share things with. Avoid those who appear to know what is best for you or who want to take control. Also beware of over-friendliness. As with all professional services, both your own as well as your practitioner's boundaries are important in this work. As the client you are going to a practitioner because they are outside your day-to-day relationships. It is a confidential setting and a space for you. It is not appropriate to get involved with the needs of your practitioner. You are paying for a professional service. This includes working in groups with a therapist as well as one-to-one work. Professional codes of practice and ethics reinforce the importance of integrity and the non-exploitation of the client. This refers both to sexuality and money. If you are unsure about the behaviour of your practitioner, around either sexuality or money, take this seriously and get advice. Unfortunately sexual abuse does occur in this profession, just as it does in all professions.

There are a number of things you may want to ask a practitioner:

- How long they have been practising their therapy and what kind of help they have been able to give to people. You may want to check their experience of a particular condition.
- What their qualifications are and where they have trained. You may also want to know who they trained with. If they are a natural healer with no formal qualifications, ask them about their experience.
- Where and how they get professional supervision or support. You may wish to check how they update their skills. The bodies of knowledge relating to the therapies described in this book are expanding rapidly and you want to know if your practitioner values being well informed and takes the necessary steps to be so.
- You may want to know if you can be assured of support from your practitioner in between sessions, especially if the effects of a treatment have been powerful for you and you

feel a little shaky emotionally or a bit worse physically. Some practitioners have phoning-in times or a cut-off time for phoning in the evening or weekends. Be clear that you know how available they may be. Obviously they have a life to lead, too, and they will need to set their boundaries around their work. All practitioners have answerphones or an answering service − if they don't then I would question their seriousness about having a professional practice − so expect to hear from them within forty-eight hours.

- Good practitioners will be clear about how they work. Some will give you an information sheet with details about the kind of contract they like to make with you, eg how long each session is, expected number of sessions, methods of payments, review sessions (to see how you are progressing or not), cancellation times and fees. If they don't have written information about these details, then it is something you might want to ask about.

- Find out where they practise from. You might want to check out transport, parking facilities, how safe you may feel in the area if you are having an evening appointment and it will be dark when you go home.

There is clearly much to think about when looking for the right therapist or practitioner. There are the practical things as well as the professional qualities of the person you go to see. You may be happy with the first person you see. If not, I believe it is worth persisting to find the person who is right for you. Often working with one therapist leads you to working with a different one later as your needs change. This depends on how far you wish to go with your own level of health and desire to grow as a person. You may simply want to deal with a symptom that is giving you pain or concern, or you may want to begin a journey of personal awakening. Whatever you choose I hope that you have a positive experience.

Part Two

The Therapies

Chapter Five
The Massage Therapies

Massage is an extension of our primitive need to touch and be touched. As said in Chapter 3, infants can die without touch. Massage helps us to relax and unwind and eases aches and pains. It triggers the release of endorphins – natural pain-killers produced by the brain – that help to block pain and produce feelings of euphoria and contentment. Massage helps us tune in to our emotional and spiritual selves.

Until the 1990s, in the UK massage had been associated almost entirely with the sex industry. It has been through the dedication of mainly female massage practitioners from the early 1980s that massage is now taken seriously. When I was first a massage practitioner in 1983 I was constantly faced with 'nudge-nudge, wink-wink' comments in social situations when I shared what my work was. The organisational work that the early pioneering professional massage associations did went a long towards changing public attitudes. We needed to define ourselves seriously and deal with issues to do with our own sexuality, so that we could be clear about how we communicated with clients and the public about our boundaries and the way in which we worked. We spent a lot of time working on codes of ethics and practice.[1] This was happening at the same time as alternative and complementary medicine was forming into a national industry. Many of us had backgrounds in local authority or health services and so could bring skills and experience to this new arena.

Massage as a therapy is very old. In China a medical treatise known as the 'Nei Ching', which is accredited to Yellow Emperor Huang-Ti, contains the earliest references to massage, three thousand years before the birth of Christ. In India, around 1800 BC, the books of the Ayur Veda refer to massage as rubbing and shampooing, which were recommended to help the body heal itself.

In ancient Greece massage was used by athletes before and after training and competing. In the *Odyssey* Homer describes how rub-downs with oil restored exhausted war heroes. Early medical literature of Egypt, Persia and Japan refer often to the benefits of massage. It was also used by the Romans. Hippocrates, Socrates and Plato are all said to have praised massage. Galen stated, 'I direct that the strokes and circuits of the hands should be made of many sorts, in order that as far as possible all muscle fibres should be rubbed in every direction.' Apparently Julius Caesar was massaged, or 'pinched', every day to help with his neuralgia.

It was unfortunate that, in the West, massage lost its popularity in the Middle Ages (tenth to fourteenth century), when there came about a general contempt of the physical body. The joy of physical well-being did not fit in with a Christian doctrine of abstinence and servitude. Previous knowledge of massage was revived during the Renaissance (fourteenth to sixteenth century). In fact many prominent physicians integrated it into their medical practices at that time.

A leap forward for massage was made by a Swedish physiologist called Per Henrik Ling. He travelled to China in the late eighteenth and early nineteenth centuries. When he returned to Sweden he combined the basic techniques he had learned with his own movements, creating an original and effective method that met more Western needs.

Currently Swedish and holistic massage and Japanese shiatsu (see Chapter 7) are probably the most popular methods in Europe and North America today:

> In the USA, at the Touch Research Institute at the University of Miami Medical School, they have found that massage can actually reduce depression. A thirty-minute neck and back massage had a pronounced effect on a wide range of patients, from anorexic and bulimic girls, abused children and adolescent mothers to psychiatric patients and those suffering from severe trauma. The effects were measurable: levels of stress-related hormones, cortisol and norepinephrine went down and the patients were more alert, less restless and more likely to sleep.[2]

Here are some other possible benefits of massage:

- chronic tension gets released, knotted tissue is eased
- helps to break down adhesions and restore strength and mobility after injury
- improves blood circulation
- improves muscle functioning because of better blood supply
- stimulates the lymphatic system, helping to eliminate waste materials
- massage of the stomach and intestines increases peristaltic movement, and aids the flow of their contents and soothes the nerves in this area. Relieves soreness and aching through removal of these waste materials
- helps maintain muscular tone and movement of bodily fluids and is good for people spending long periods of time in a bed or wheelchair
- helps through passive stretching when a person is unable to take exercise
- improves circulation to joints and therefore helps to relieve inflammation/pain of arthritis
- helps with pain control

- helps to clear nasal congestion/sinus problems
- relieves headaches
- relieves back pain
- can bring a feeling of wholeness
- may heighten awareness and put person in touch with her/his 'real' self
- can encourage trust, empathy and respect
- can bring deep relaxation leading to physical and psychological well-being
- can bring renewed energy
- can clear the mind
- can help improve self-esteem
- generally feels really good!

Massage is often used in conjunction with OSTEOPATHY or CHIROPRACTIC to help re-establish and maintain the postural alignment of the body.

There are many different types of massage, including SWEDISH, INTUITIVE, INFANT MASSAGE, HEAD AND FACIAL MASSAGE, MASSAGE FOR THE ELDERLY, REMEDIAL AND SPORTS MASSAGE. In Yorkshire there is now training in EQUINE MASSAGE. Apparently horses respond really positively. You can massage your pets. (You can also give hands-on healing to animals; see Chapter 8.) These forms of massage originate from many different parts of the world, including Sweden, Tibet, Thailand, Russia, Japan, India and Esalen (California, US).

Massage is also used increasingly in hospices and hospitals, for cardiac, cancer and psychiatric patients. Together with the use of aromatherapy, practitioners are making significant inroads into being part of conventional health care.[3]

Contraindications

There are general contraindications to most forms of massage; that is, times when it should not be given. It should be avoided during acute periods of inflammation of skin or joints or if you have infective skin conditions such as scabies, ringworm or athlete's foot. There should be no strong pressure or percussive movements during pregnancy and only very light stroking movements for varicose veins or recent scars or wounds from surgery.

I have chosen to describe here some of the main types of massage. To explore this field further please turn to the bibliography.

Swedish massage

The aim of Swedish massage is to maintain or restore good health through specific and careful manipulation of joints and muscles. It can be broken down into four main movements:

- Effleurage: long strokes, using the flat of the hand, which soothe and relax. Effleurage is used at the beginning and end of a massage and in between deeper, more specific work in the tissues and joints. It helps to spread the oil or cream you may be using and helps to build up trust between client and practitioner. During the effleuraging the practitioner can feel where particular areas of tension are. It relaxes the surface muscles and prepares them for stronger, deeper movements. It can be wonderful to be simply effleuraged all over (omitting parts that you may not want touched).

- Petrissage: this involves kneading – taking large muscles into the hands and kneading, rather like you do with bread dough; rolling and gently squeezing the tissues.

- Friction: this is small circular movements used on tissues pressed deeply against the bone. The practitioner applies this pressure around joints, working on bands of connective tissue, ie tendons, ligaments, fascia and joint capsules. The intention is to release specific areas of tension and blockage.

- Tapotement: these are stimulating movements that are designed to tone and strengthen muscles. Cupping and hacking are two of the main movements and are called percussion.

Holistic massage

The holistic massage practitioner is generally someone who has trained in Swedish massage but whose training has incorporated a broader view of the human body-mind. They will be as concerned about the psychological and spiritual benefits as they will the physical. They are likely to have been introduced to the subtle energy bodies and so will be working with the energy flows that can be sensed through the hands on and off the body, as well as with muscle, tissue and bone.

Holistic massage tends to be much more gentle than other forms of massage, although you should still feel satisfaction from having indepth touch. It is important to feel those painful spots which I call 'good hurts'. The right pressure relieves all sorts of sore places.

Holistic massage practitioners may well play relaxation music while they work. However it is preferable that they ask you beforehand if you would like this. They may also burn a candle, and/or aromatherapy oils to add to the healing quality of the environment. The whole emphasis of this kind of massage is that the person feels she is being nurtured and supported. The room should obviously be clean and also be private, warm and with dim lighting. Such an environment is aimed at helping people feel emotionally safe and avoids appearing too much like a medical clinic.

Harriet is English, white, single and is a publishing editor. Here is her contribution:

'My initial symptom was precise back pain but I soon realised that I needed massage regularly as a way to reduce stress. I felt I was holding a lot of tension physically. I had just come out of a long-term relationship that had put me through enormous emotional stress.

The first massage I received was very cathartic. I experienced intense heat sensation in the small of my back and deep relaxation, which actually culminated in my weeping. I was not aware on an intellectual level of thinking about my inner turmoil, but felt rather that the tears had sprung up as a release system rather than on account of any specific unhappy thoughts.

In the early days of my receiving massage each session would have an enormous effect on me. I would either feel tremendously invigorated or deeply relaxed. Clearly I was taking the most from the sessions when I needed it most. Now, some three years later, I still find my massage sessions a great help for grounding and relaxing myself physically, but my experiences on the massage table are less heightened.'

My own story of massage shows how it helped me recover from bulimia nervosa, and led me into doing more psychotherapy for myself:

In 1982 a close friend and I went to a Swedish massage course together. She had a problem with her feet. They hadn't grown properly and she had big bunions, with her toes squashed into a triangle shape. Her feet sometimes ached and her doctor had recommended an operation that would involve breaking the toes and resetting them. We decided to help each other with massage. She later decided against an operation. She helped me with the bulimia and the disgust I felt at the time towards the shape of my belly. After a few practice sessions when she massaged me there I started belching, almost uncontrollably. She responded naturally by stroking my back. I wanted to curl up, which she allowed me to do. Very soon she was behaving like a mother winding a baby. I regressed into a deep, early place in myself. I felt I was remembering my early babyhood. I felt I was receiving substitute mothering for what my own mother was unable to do at the time.

After a couple of sessions like this we realised that we were getting out of depth in our friendship. So I went into therapy for the second time and worked with a neo-Reichian therapist for two years. Amongst other things this kind of therapy encouraged regression work through contact with the body. I worked through a great deal of stored-up pain and memories concerning the first few weeks of my life. It was invaluable.

Sports and remedial massage

People who do a lot of sport, dance or rigorous exercise may sustain injury to their bones, joints and muscles, tendons and ligaments. When there is an obvious structural or mechanical cause to a problem then a structural or mechanical form of massage is what is needed. Physical therapy in this sense is akin to traditional PHYSIOTHERAPY. In fact physiotherapists originally were massage practitioners. The massage aspect of the work lost its emphasis when medical technology and equipment became the norm. Many physiotherapists have returned to learn more about massage and other forms of bodywork.[4]

Sports massage is also used as part of the athletes' training programme, supporting them to reach their physical potential. Mel Cash states, 'Some athletes may be tempted to take steroids because it is expected to enable them to increase the quality and quantity of their training. Massage could help achieve this safely and legally.'[5]

Sports massage is very anatomically based, with touch techniques that go deeply into the joints and muscles. They are based on the Swedish strokes already mentioned with possible additions such as rocking and shaking. The practitioner will have extensive knowledge of sports injuries, which arise from overuse and extending the limits of the body. Before an event, massage can help an athlete fine tune his or her body and tissues can be prepared for the stresses he or she is about to undergo. The general warm-up and warm-down exercises that sports people need to do can be enhanced by the use of massage, with particular muscles being focused on.

Acute injuries such as strains and sprains are most commonly experienced by athletes. A strain to a muscle or tendon is when the tissue fibres become torn or damaged. This causes bleeding and swelling. As well as pain and dysfunction, heat and redness may be noticed if the injury is near the surface. A sprain is when some or all the fibres of a ligament supporting a joint are torn, and this happens when a joint is forced beyond its normal range. Here the swelling and bruising is considerable with a lot of pain and dysfunction. The practitioner will advise the person to rest, apply ice (which helps reduce the swelling by slowing down the blood circulation), compress the injury with a firm pad strapped in place, and elevate the area as much as possible. This allows gravity to help reduce the swelling. The practitioner will not massage the injury directly, but massage other parts of the body, which can help improve lymphatic drainage. The practitioner will have knowledge of chronic injuries such as bone fractures of different kinds, inflammation of tendons, dislocated joints, muscle and ligament injuries.

My own current massage practitioner works with remedial massage. The techniques she uses, which are particularly beneficial to me for joint and muscle pain, are called muscle energy techniques. These techniques are manipulative movements in which the client actively uses her muscles from a controlled position in a specific direction against a distinct counter-force supplied by the practitioner. I have experienced immediate pain relief from receiving this technique. These techniques are called isometric and isotonic (6) and some of their uses are: to strengthen weak muscles, stretch tight muscles and fascia, improve blood circulation to the area and help mobilise joints where movement is restricted.

Another technique used for releasing muscle spasms resulting from traumas, such as stiff neck from whiplash or muscle spasm in the back, is called strain-counterstrain. Where tension and pain will increase if stretching is attempted, instead the muscle is shortened by gently moving it further in the direction of the contraction until it feels comfortable. As the client you do not use any effort yourself but rather allow your practitioner to move the relevant part of your body. This position is then held for over a minute during which time the nerves in the muscle that control tension can calm and thus stop the spasm. The muscle then can be very carefully and slowly passively stretched beyond its previously restricted range. This new position then needs to be held for another minute to allow the tissues and nervous system to adapt. This takes skill and knowledge because the practitioner needs to understand the nature of the muscles involved.

Indian head massage

Indian head massage has been popular throughout the Indian subcontinent for over a thousand years and is practised mainly by women. It includes massage of the scalp, face (including the ears), neck, shoulders, upper back and upper arms. The work is very thorough and precise. Many different techniques are employed, using the thumbs, fingertips and pads, heel of the hand and the whole of the hands. The practitioner follows a set sequence using sweeping, pulling, pushing, squeezing and rolling movements over muscles and bone.

'Ironing down' is a smooth, firm stroke used across the shoulders and down the arms. 'Ruffling' is very light 'shampooing' movements all over the head. 'Tapping and hacking' is rhythmically done over the head. Gentle pressure points are administered to the face. Sometimes the techniques are gentle, sometimes much more vigorous. The first part of the sequence is stimulating. This is followed by relaxation and healing. The healing aspect involves work with the CHAKRAS at the crown, third eye (middle of forehead) and throat (see Chapter 8). Sometimes special oils are used to nourish the hair roots, which helps improve the texture of the hair, possibly even reducing hair loss.

By stimulating scalp circulation, this form of massage relaxes the scalp and tones up the subcutaneous muscles, relieving eye strain and headaches and improving concentration. It also can help with muscle tension and joint movement as it involves stretching and mobilising the tissues of the neck and shoulders. In the workplace it is especially helpful to computer users and, of course, there is no need to undress for this treatment.

Receiving Indian head massage for me has been memorable. Having every millimetre of my head, neck and shoulders worked on was exceptionally pleasant and mentally calming. It was the detail and thoroughness of the touch that impressed me.

This is the kind of massage that women, and men, can learn to give to one another, as indeed women in India have been doing for centuries.

Infant massage

Infant massage is an ancient tradition in some cultures. It had not been practised widely in the West until a woman called Vimala Schnieder McLure founded the International Association of Infant Massage (IAIM) in the United States. Vimala had worked in India during the 1970s and had learned about infant massage there. She observed that even the most poverty-stricken mothers massaged their babies as part of a daily routine. After returning home and having her own children Vimala developed a massage sequence specially for babies. She based this on the strokes she had observed in India, and added elements of SWEDISH MASSAGE, REFLEXOLOGY and YOGA.

The UK chapter of the IAIM was set up in July 1997 (see Resources). Its vision is that by promoting and teaching infant massage it will become a parenting tradition throughout the world, helping future generations to express more compassion towards and responsibility for their fellow human beings.

The benefits of infant massage are fourfold:

1. Bonding: attachment and interaction.
2. Relaxation: for both parents and babies. This can improve the baby's sleep patterns.
3. Stimulation: of the baby's respiratory, immune, digestive, circulatory and eliminatory systems.
4. Relief: from colic, wind, constipation and mucous.

Aromatherapy

Many massage practitioners go on to study aromatherapy. The combination of a deeply relaxing massage and the use of essential oils enhances the overall effectiveness of the treatment. The addition of essential oils into a base or carrier oil facilitates absorption into the bloodstream and tissues via the skin. Olfactory nerve endings in the nose pick up neuro-chemical messages and these are passed to the limbic area of the brain. Here they quickly affect our emotions and moods. Chemical changes in the body can include the release of encephalins and endorphins, the body's natural painkillers.

Here I am focusing more directly on the use of essential oils in massage. However, they may also be used in baths, steam inhalation and oil burners. It should be noted that there is a great difference between using aromatherapy generally and using it clinically; that is, using the oils for specific symptom relief. For more serious conditions you really need to contact a clinical aromatherapist. General applications are fine for self-help where general relaxation is required. Even so, you need to study the different healing qualities of each oil.

When using essential oils there needs to be an awareness of storing them safely – in a cool, dark place, keeping them out of the reach of children and in dark glass bottles. To benefit from the therapeutic properties buying a high quality oil is essential and will be reflected in the price that you pay for them. Careful use of the oils can be of great benefit for a wide range of women's health conditions.

Aromatherapy is the use of oils extracted from plants. In massage they are added in small amounts (one or a few drops) to a base or carrier oil. The carrier oil, such as almond, avocado, wheatgerm, grapeseed or sesame, provides lubrication and also dilutes the essential oils. Usually three to six drops of the essential oil is added to ten millilitres of the carrier oil (approximately two to three per cent). Often ten per cent of wheatgerm oil is added as a natural preservative if larger amounts are made to be kept.

The use of aromatic oils dates back at least as far as ancient Egypt with their use in mummification and for purifying the air. The Greeks also practised aromatherapy. Hippocrates said in the fourth century BC, 'The way to health is to have an aromatic bath and scented massage every day.' Today it is well known by chemists that these oils have antibacterial and anti-viral properties. They can also be antiseptic, analgesic, expectorant, diuretic, antidepressant, antispasmodic, and can aid digestion and circulation.

Modern aromatherapy is said to have begun with the research of a French chemist called Rene Maurice Gattefossé, who also coined the term aromatherapy. He burned his hand in his family's perfume factory and plunged it into a container of lavender oil. Within hours his hand had healed with no scarring or infection. He went on to develop the use of essential oils in dermatology.

There are around three hundred essential oils used today, obtained from many parts of plants such as flowers, roots, fruit, seeds, bark, twigs and leaves. Different processes are used to extract the oils, one of which is steam or water distillation. Here steam or boiling water is passed through the plant material, which gives up its oil. The mixture that results is then passed through a cooling chamber and the water and oil collected. The oil is drawn off, and the water may be sold as floral water, or recycled.

Carole is forty and the mother of two. Here is her story about aromatherapy. It highlights the value and importance of having your GP's support when receiving non-conventional treatment. It also illustrates how important it is for comple-mentary practitioners to have appropriate communication skills.

'I found myself suffering from the second bout of severe clinical depression in two years. I previously was prescribed antidepressant tablets, the side-effects of which I found difficult to handle. So this time I was keen to find an alternative method of seeing this period through to a satisfactory conclusion.

My doctor at the time was very approachable and open minded. Together, we decided that, with her supervision, I would undertake to have regular aromatherapy treatments instead of a prescription of antidepressants. Because of the likelihood of feeling suicidal through the depression we agreed that I would visit her once a week during the treatments so that she could monitor the situation.

The fact that I was seeing my doctor made me feel that I was not taking any undue risks with my health. It was important to me to have that safety net. I would not have undertaken using aromatherapy alone unless I had had the support of my doctor.

The aromatherapist and I chose the essential oils together for each session depending on how I was feeling that particular day. We used different combinations of sandalwood, frankincense, grapefruit, bergamot, rosemary, basil and neroli over a period of fifteen sessions.

Receiving treatments from a sympathetic therapist, someone that was prepared to listen to how I felt, combined with the properties of the essential oils, was indeed a very nurturing experience for me. I found that after the massage I wanted to talk and having a therapist with good counselling skills to listen was just what I needed.

Resting as much as I needed after each treatment gave my body the opportunity to heal. The first treatment was marked by the fact that I could hardly bear to be touched as I was so exhausted and fragile, and by the fifteenth session I felt well enough to go onto monthly treatments.'

Although oils are available in chemists, gift shops and even market stalls, the quality of these oils varies considerably. Some can be very toxic if used wrongly. I have selected just a few of the properties of the oils. To use them effectively you need a more exhaustive list of their properties.[7] If you have a serious medical condition or complex health problem it is important that you seek the advice of a professional aromatherapist, preferably with the support of your medical doctor as well.

Some of the oils can be grouped as follows (using two to six drops per ten millilitres of base oil):

- Those that relax and are sedatives, eg lavender, chamomile, sandalwood and marjoram. Lavender is good for burns, headaches, insomnia and panic attacks. It is one of the few oils that can be used neat (1 or 2 drops). Roman chamomile can be added for insomnia and is also good for eczema and dry skin. German chamomile is excellent for inflammation. Marjoram can also be added to lavender for insomnia. It is antispasmodic, used for digestive and respiratory spasms, as found in irritable bowel syndrome and tickly coughs. For persistent and irritating coughs use sandalwood.

- Those that stimulate, eg tea-tree, juniper and rosemary. Rosemary helps concentration, and in massage or in the bath can energise and ease muscle pain. Tea-tree is really good for colds, flu and infections. It is also a strong antifungal agent and is used to relieve athlete's foot. Juniper is renowned for its diuretic property, making it the ideal choice for cystitis.

- Those that regulate and balance, eg geranium, rosewood and frankincense. Geranium helps balance skin that is either too dry or too oily, and can also help with PMT and irregular periods. Rosewood is a good choice for anyone with lowered immunity or chronic fatigue. Frankincense has a meditative quality, and is used for stretch marks and mature, dry skin.

Pregnancy and childbirth

The use of aromatherapy during pregnancy and childbirth can have great benefits, helping you to relax, cope better with labour and to bond with your baby. Using essential oils at this time must be done with due consideration to the changes that are taking place in your body. For this reason there are a variety of oils that are not appropriate to use at this time and professional advice really must be sought.[8]

General **pregnancy massage**, without necessarily the use of aromatherapy oils, is invaluable. It may help relieve morning sickness, fatigue, backache and cramps, anxiety and fluid retention. It helps to tone and strengthen your body. It supports you in preparing for the labour, giving you a nurturing time for yourself. It encourages you to relax and have a positive attitude.

Stephen Fulder refers to a six-month pilot study at the John Radcliffe Hospital in Oxford, in which various essential oils were used clinically with 585 women in labour. Lavender was used for anxiety and pain, peppermint for nausea and vomiting, and clary sage to increase contractions. 'The programme was a great success, and mothers reported a high degree of satisfaction and relief.'[9]

Out of all the bodywork therapies available at the time of writing, aromatherapy, along with reflexology, has captured the public's imagination and has been accepted by the medical profession within both primary and hospital care as very respectable. Many nurses have trained in these therapies from their own interest.

A word of warning
There are serious concerns expressed by professional aromatherapists about the unsafe use of essential oils by the general public. Because of their popularity, commercial interest

in essential oils has meant that oils of dubious quality are on the market. In shops and marketplaces they are often not kept in a cool, dark place, may not be labelled properly and may not be sold in proper dropper bottles that are essential for accurate dispensing.

Contraindications

Don't use undiluted oils directly on the skin, except for lavender and tea-tree, or over any skin infection, recent wounds or inflammation. Care should be taken over your choice of oils if you suffer from high blood pressure, asthma, epilepsy or sensitive skin. If you are trying to get pregnant, or wish to use oils on children, seek further advice. Some oils like bergamot, for example, are photosensitive and therefore should not be used before going out into direct sunlight.

When choosing base or carrier oil do note that some are nut- or wheat-based and therefore should not be used if you are allergic to either.

Some oils, such as eucalyptus and peppermint, can counteract the effects of homoeopathic remedies, so it is wise to avoid these if you are receiving homoeopathy. Speak to your homoeopath as opinions vary.

General contraindications for massage include where there is infectious disease, deep vein thrombosis, inflammation, and soon after surgery.

Self-help

You can easily massage yourself. Although it is not quite as enjoyable as being massaged by someone else, you can help yourself soothe away tension. You can energise yourself before beginning your day, or you can use slow strokes to unwind in the evening. You can massage your own hands or feet. I sometimes do my feet while I'm watching the television. You need to be comfortable. You can work through clothes, but use oil if you are working on bare skin. You can use a body lotion, although this gets absorbed into the skin quickly. Here is a simple sequence for massaging your shoulders. It will help relax you and can help prevent headaches. You can do it through your clothes or on bare skin.

1. Stroke your left shoulder with your right hand all the way from the base of your skull, down the side of your neck, across your shoulder and down off your arm and hand. Repeat this a few times, and then do it on the other side.
2. Using your right hand knead your left shoulder by squeezing and releasing the flesh at the top of your back as it becomes your shoulder. You can use your fingertips to work deeply into the tense muscle. Repeat on the other shoulder with your left hand.
3. Make your right hand into a fist shape and pound your left shoulder. Keep your wrist flexible. Repeat on the other side with your left hand.
4. Repeat number 1.

You can also help relieve a tension headache:
1. Add a drop of lavender oil to a carrier oil and massage over your temples and forehead.
2. Using the ball of your thumb or fingers press firmly along under the base of your skull from ear to ear. Press and rotate into each of the hollows. When you come to a sore spot work around it and then into it gently and firmly until the soreness eases.

Please note: the causes of headaches can be complex, including psychological upset, toxicity, irregularities in the blood vessels as well as general tension and stress. If you have persistent headaches seek professional help.

Chapter Six

Manipulation Therapies and Postural Education

The manipulation therapies are concerned primarily with the spine, although techniques overlap with other therapies and the effects are wide reaching. The most established therapies – OSTEOPATHY and CHIROPRACTIC – focus on the skeletal structure. Others – THE BOWEN TECHNIQUE and ROLFING, POSTURAL INTEGRATION and Hellerwork – focus on the fascial structure. Fascia is the connective tissue found throughout the body. It covers all of the muscles, organs, nerves, blood vessels and cells of the body. Myofascia is the fascia that covers the muscles and shapes, supports and separates them.

Most people go to an osteopath or chiropractor because of back or neck pain. This can often be a way in to other therapies and lifestyle changes. Often people turn to these therapies when standard physiotherapy hasn't helped sufficiently.

Care needs to be taken as to who you go to, as these skeletal manipulative therapies are more invasive than general touch therapies and mistakes can aggravate the condition. However, training is generally long and demanding. Always check the credentials of a practitioner.

Although I have emphasised the structural, bony nature of the skeletal therapies, they can also sometimes affect the receiver in deeply psychological and energetic ways, as is discussed towards the end of the chapter under ROLFING.

Osteopathy

The founder of osteopathy was Dr Andrew Taylor Still, a mid-Western American of the nineteenth century. He was a medical doctor, healer and minister and, after the death of three of his children because of viral meningitis, he turned to the Hippocratic idea that the cure of disease lies within the body itself. He had also studied engineering and believed that for the body to function well its different parts had to move freely. He became convinced that a lot of injury and illness was caused by tension in muscles and bones that were badly aligned and this poor alignment was the result of chronic bad posture, previous physical injuries and emotional stresses. Through adjusting the framework of the body its internal systems would function better.

Osteopathy is a system of manipulation to bring the structure of the body back into balance. Its basic theory is that structure determines function. Osteopathic treatment changes the way the bones of the body relate to each other, freeing obstructions between joints and so improving well-being. Osteopaths work directly with bony structure throughout the body.

Benefits
Osteopathy works particularly well for:

- acute or chronic back and neck pain
- all muscular and joint pain
- sports and other injuries
- arthritic and rheumatic conditions
- headaches
- digestive problems
- PMS.

The osteopath will observe the patient's range of movement, standing, sitting and lying, and then apply a variety of treatment techniques using her hands. These can include soft tissue stretching and joint movements: rhythmic and gentle, or high-velocity thrust techniques (the well-known 'crunches' and 'clicks'). These all improve mobility and range of movement of the joints. If you are nervous of having parts of your spine manipulated (clicked, cracked or crunched a little) then you may prefer CRANIAL OSTEOPATHY, CRANIO-SACRAL THERAPY, ZERO BALANCING or McTIMONEY CHIROPRACTIC.

Treatment usually involves undressing down to underwear and sessions can last from thirty to sixty minutes, the first session being longer to allow time for a medical history to be taken. One session may be all that is required to give pain relief and required mobility but usually a series of six or more treatments is necessary. As with other therapies, if you have back weakness or joint problems, seeing an osteopath regularly, ie once a month, is invaluable for maintenance and prevention.

Contraindications

It is important to go to a reputable osteopath as, although a correct manipulation can feel like a miracle in pain relief, an incorrect one can make things worse. Osteopathy is not recommended for osteoporosis (loss of density in the bone, often due to wear and tear) and where the joints are inflamed.

Harriet was quoted in the section about holistic massage. She uses osteopathy as well:

'I first saw an osteopath on the recommendation of my masseuse since a particular problem felt bone-related rather than muscle-related. I have had very positive responses to treatment...I have found an excellent practitioner...She has used both high-velocity thrust and gentle manipulation on me and I always find her treatment extremely helpful. The high-velocity thrusts work particularly well on me and I have never experienced any pain with them.

I would definitely recommend osteopathy as a form of treatment but say this with caution as I have heard of people having bad experiences. I would recommend seeing someone on recommendation. As a woman I would prefer to be treated by a woman (and this goes for massage too)...

Having regular body work has also taught me to think more carefully about how I carry my body, sit, lift things, etc. I have also learned to recognise the need for rest, good diet and regular exercise.'

Cranial osteopathy

I have been extremely fortunate in having been treated by excellent cranial osteopaths and I highly rate this therapy for back and neck pain, headaches, digestive problems, and during pregnancy. It is very useful in conjunction with counselling or psychotherapy.

Until the early part of this century it was believed that the skull – the sixteen bones of the cranium and face – was fixed and that there was nothing that could be manipulated. However, William Garner Sutherland, a trained osteopath, found that there were minute movements taking place in the sutures of the skull that, just like other joints, could be gently manipulated back into balance. He also discovered rhythms that could be detected within the cranium.

There is a kind of pulse that echoes the fluctuation of the cerebrospinal fluid (this is a liquid that bathes the tissues of the spinal cord and the brain). In a healthy adult this should pulse at ten to fourteen beats a minute. This optimum level is not reached when someone is ill or has a problem. By gently manipulating both the cranium and the sacrum the pulse can be corrected. The osteopath's sense of touch is used to identify and correct these slight disturbances of tissue mobility and fluid flow, not only in the skull, but throughout the whole body.

Benefits
Cranial osteopathy can help relieve:

- different types of head pain, including sinusitis and migraine, as well as the after-effects of head injuries such as whiplash and dental work
- circulation problems
- high blood pressure
- stomach ulcers
- disturbances of balance
- breathing difficulties.

Benefits for children
Because of its gentleness, cranial osteopathy is very good for children. Many kinds of conditions are treatable. Here are a few:

- postural problems
- knock knees
- glue ear
- sleep problems
- difficult behaviour such as head banging, exaggerated aggression
- stress problems that may be associated with high expectations at school, such as tense shoulders, headaches, stomach pains
- children with learning difficulties, including autistic children. In these cases outcomes of treatment can range from phenomenal success to no real obvious improvement.

Benefits of osteopathy and cranial osteopathy during pregnancy and after the birth
Many osteopaths, especially those also trained in cranial osteopathy, specialise in treating pregnant women, babies and

children. Pregnant women can get help with symptoms such as morning sickness, tiredness and problems with the sacralo-iliac joint in the pelvis.

If the baby's position is causing discomfort the osteopath may work, for example, with the mother's pelvis to relieve pressure on a nerve root and make more space for the baby to shift around. Working with the lymphatic draining in the pelvis can help prevent common pregnancy problems such as varicose veins and haemorrhoids (piles). Osteopathy can also help the mother emotionally. Sometimes she may be resisting the pregnancy on some level and treatment can help her to integrate the experience of her body being pregnant with her mind.

Newborn babies, as well as their mothers, can be treated to help them recover from the trauma of birth, especially if it has been a difficult one. Mother and baby can be in shock. The cranial osteopath will often work with mother and baby as one unit. Such treatment can help with the bonding between them; a kind of energetic shift can take place for the mother while her baby is receiving treatment. If the baby has been in a special care unit the mother may have held back the bonding process because she is afraid she will lose her child. As the mother lets go of this fear, so the baby too can relax and their bond can be created.

Physical difficulties in newborns, such as distorted or squashed heads and colic, can be treated with cranial osteopathy.

I personally would like to see every newborn baby be given cranial osteopathy as a matter of course, as long as their parents agreed. I believe it would give the child a wonderful start in life and mean that their brain and general functioning would begin in balance.

Lydia is single, in her mid-thirties, and is a management consultant. She went for treatment because she had neck and shoulder/upper back tension. Here is her story:

'The first time I went to my cranial osteopath I lay on the table feeling completely duped, while she placed her hands on different parts of me, often seeming to hold them there for a long time. I felt really foolish and I thought that I was being completely ripped off. I was thinking, I could do this myself at home for free. She talked about there being less energy in the left side of my body. I thought, How on earth can she tell that? I am wasting £40!

After she finished she asked me to get up and walk around and see how I felt. I stood up and walked and I was astounded. My left shoulder, which had bothered me for years, felt free and light. I had never before understood when people spoke of feeling lighter in their bodies. Now I did. I have been transformed from being a disbelieving cynic to being curious and fascinated about the "energies" with which my cranial osteopath works.'

Here is the story of a single mother, who is in her early forties and comes from a large Anglo–Irish Catholic, working–class family:

'I have experienced a range of body therapies mainly because of my disability. At eight weeks old I had meningitis. I survived with a weakness to my left-side limbs. I went to a swimming club for handicapped children from three to thirteen years old. At sixteen surgery was offered but declined by my mum. I was dismissed from the children's hospital as the adults considered my development had been remarkable, considering. I just had to live with it.

At twenty-five years old I met another woman with a similar disability. It was then that I realised that I was so used to pain that I didn't even mention it. My left leg is shorter than the right, putting strain on my toes, ankle, knee, pelvis and back. There is bone and muscle atrophy, and nerve damage creating heightened sensitivity and immobility of my left foot. My friend recommended a cranial osteopath.

I have worked with one woman for years. At first I needed regular treatments...over about eighteen months. Then I would go about every three to four months for maintenance. Then as I wanted. I still go back occasionally. These treatments helped a great deal.'

It was through osteopathy with cranial osteopathy that I began my recovery after my spinal injury:

In 1979 at the age of thirty I fractured my sacrum in a roller-skating accident. I was on a roller rink which was was full; there were families, teenagers, friends, disco dancers. I remember thinking to myself, It is very crowded, someone is going to get hurt; I'll go round one more time and then I'll get off. What I didn't realise was that this inner voice was referring to me. In that 'one more time' I was knocked down by someone coming up behind me, and I landed on the base of my spine. The pain was excruciating. A couple of people rescued me and dragged me to the side of the rink, where I promptly felt very sick and passed out.

I was in chronic lower-back pain for around eighteen months with very little relief. Through a close friend, I was fortunate enough to hear about a cranial osteopath, who was a fourth-year student at the European School of Osteopathy in Maidstone, Kent. This meant I could have treatment at low cost, which was important because I was living on Invalidity Benefit. At the first session I was given homoeopathy as well (hypericum for injury to the spine and arnica for shock).

Receiving cranial osteopathy was like coming two hundred years forward in time compared to the approach of the orthopaedic doctors. I found the bodywork fascinating. I could feel all sorts of sensations throughout my body as the osteopath gently and carefully altered the shape of my spine. Unbeknown to me I had a scoliosis — a sideways curvature — in my upper back and the trauma at the base had shown up the weaknesses further up the spine. I knew my posture wasn't that good, but now it mattered a lot because I was finding it difficult holding myself up for any length of time without severe lower-back pain. During the sessions I learned how quickly my body responded to the treatment and for the first time in my life I felt affirmed for my sensitivity. I learned I could view my sensitivity as a gift rather than a burden.

After nine months or so my mobility very much improved. But I was still in too much pain to get back to work on a regular basis. My osteopath invited me to be treated by his teacher, at the European College. The osteopathic teacher gave a lecture about my back; he treated me, lying on a treatment couch, in a classroom. The language was so technical and so impressed me that I began a new belief in the efficacy of the treatment. Although I had trusted my own osteopath and the treatment before, it was so new to me, so different from hospitals and doctors, that part of me wasn't sure about it. Now that I was introduced to a training school I was taken with the professionalism and science of it all. At that first session he simply moved something very gently in between my shoulder blades. Over the following two days I felt a lot of movement in my back and knew that I had begun a new level of healing. The next session involved a manipulation to my neck. Afterwards I literally felt as if my head was screwed on more correctly. I could see more clearly. The teacher then supervised my osteopath for a few sessions back in London.

I remember one session when I had by now been quite free of pain for a few days, but had felt extremely depressed. I would be on a bus and be fighting back streams of tears. I had no idea what it was about. When I shared this with the osteopaths they seemed unsurprised. The teacher then touched my sacrum (the first time since the accident), making a little 'ping' movement. I felt the sensation of the depression slowly move up my spine, right up out of my head. I couldn't believe it! The experience of depression seemed directly related to energy locked in my sacrum. I got back to work and continued the osteopathy on and off for the next fifteen years. I used it to maintain my health and prevent chronic back pain, and still have a session from time to time.

Cranio-sacral therapy

Based on the same premise that restrictions of the cranio-sacral rhythm can cause health problems, this method of bodywork developed out of cranial osteopathy. However, practitioners do not need training in osteopathy. There is some contention about this in the osteopathic profession as the training for cranio-sacral therapy is less demanding and there are concerns that unintended harm could be done. This is difficult to assess, especially as so much seems to depend on the practitioner as a person, as well as their skills and techniques. A cranio-sacral therapist may often be better trained in cranial techniques than a general osteopath.

This description of cranio-sacral therapy equally applies to cranial osteopathy. The idea that traumatic experiences get 'locked up' into the body's tissues runs through most of the bodywork therapies. It follows that these patterns of stored traumas can restrict the body's easy functioning and can give rise to problems as the years go by. Since these involve emotional issues as well, this therapy is a good adjunct, but *not* a replacement for psychotherapy.

Like cranial osteopathy, the actual treatment is extremely gentle and uses no manipulation. The receiver remains clothed and usually lies on a treatment table. The therapist uses a very light touch on the head and other areas, such as the sacrum.

She 'listens' to the patterns of subtle energy or fluid movement in the body. The body recognises its own patterns of barriers, which then release, and the body continues on with its own healing process. As with cranial osteopathy, cranio-sacral therapy follows the pace set by your own body. So you stay comfortable and in control. As you become more and more relaxed you may become aware of many sensations and sometimes old symptoms recur briefly as tensions are released. Sometimes there are spontaneous movements or twitching.

Because it is so noninvasive it is safe and suitable for people of all ages, and can help with practically any condition, especially where greater mobility, calmness and well-being are sought.

Benefits
A wide range of conditions may respond favourably such as:

- headaches and migraines
- digestive disorders
- jaw problems
- back pain
- hormonal imbalances
- insomnia
- tinnitus
- joint pains.

You may feel you have nothing wrong with you but benefit nevertheless, because this kind of deep relaxation helps you let go of unconscious tensions, so you are actually releasing any potential problem before it arises.

Contraindications
There can be some concern that, because cranio-sacral therapists do not complete the same depth and length of medical training as osteopaths and cranial osteopaths, they may

be dealing with severe symptoms inappropriately. The whole ethos is that the practitioner believes that the client's body has within it the wisdom to solve its own problems and that sensitivity, dedication, caring and patience are the major prerequisites of the practitioner's skills. So it focuses very much on the process of healing. My opinion is that a therapy should minimise the description of medical symptoms that it can help with. Although many medical symptoms may indeed be helped, expectations of specific physical improvement from the client's point of view need to be kept realistic. This point is relevant to all the more subtle, light-touch therapies.

In my view there is a definite overlap between cranial work – cranial osteopathy or cranio-sacral therapy – and LAYING ON HAND HEALING. The experience and quality of light touch is similar, as is the contact with the individual's subtle energetic rhythm. However, the cranio-sacral therapist or the cranial osteopath will be working with a deep knowledge of the tissues and fascia beneath her hands, something that a laying on hands healer may not have or need to have. Although it is unknown as yet how cranio-sacral therapy works precisely, the treatment is based upon known anatomy and physiology. On a personal note I have found it to be one of the most deeply relaxing therapies I have experienced.

Chiropractic

The aim of the chiropractor is to correct joint misalignment, particularly of the spine, using manipulation. By manipulating and mobilising the joints and soft tissues the treatment aims to restore the normal movement, and therefore relieve strain and stress to the joints and nerves of the spine. When normal balance is achieved, the body is able to use its own healing mechanism to correctly repair as much damaged tissue as possible. When vertebrae are out of alignment the potential for nerve interference, or 'subluxation', is considerable.[1]

As with all the manipulative therapies, this differs from the traditional medical approach of bedrest with anti-inflammatory and painkilling medication, which potentially hides the symptoms and allows scar tissue to develop. This is not to say that painkillers aren't sometimes necessary. They help us cope, and relief from pain usually relaxes the affected muscles, but their effects should not be regarded as a 'cure'.

Chiropractic began in 1895 with Daniel David Palmer in Iowa. He was a healer who learned that the ancient Egyptians had known how to replace displaced vertebrae and that Hippocrates had also used manipulation of the spine to give relief to a wide range of illnesses; this was the art of 'bone setting'. It has also long been an important part of Chinese medicine. Palmer developed the theory that all disease could be caused by impingement on the nerves as they leave the spine. He put vertebrae back into position and a man's hearing returned; another's heart trouble miraculously cured. Chiropractic came to Britain before the First World War.

In 1991 the British Medical Research Council trial proved chiropractic treatment significantly more effective for patients with chronic and severe back pain than outpatient medical/physiotherapy treatment. In 1994 the Consumer Standards Advisory Group recommended that GPs refer back-pain sufferers to chiropractors for effective treatment.

A treatment involves the chiropractor taking a detailed history to assess the possible causes of your complaint. A thorough chiropractic examination – the unique skill of a trained chiropractor – involves feeling the joint movement and location of the bones of the spine to determine which alignments and movements are abnormal. During an adjustment the chiropractor applies a small force to the problematic bone in a brisk, specific thrust. Sometimes a small 'popping' sound is heard similar to the sound made by someone 'cracking' their knuckles. This is the joint fluid releasing gas into the joint, and is usually painless.

MASSAGE is also often part of the treatment, relaxing the muscles first so that making adjustment is easy and pain-free. Advice is also given on exercise, stretching, posture, ergonomics and diet. The length of treatment obviously varies according to your condition and age and any aggravating factors, such as your occupation. There is an initial phase – usually two or three treatments – aimed at relieving the immediate symptoms, then a rehabilitation phase, perhaps four more treatments, for the joints to be 'educated' to function normally. There is then a maintenance phase; a treatment every month or quarter to help keep the spine stable. This is preventative care and helps stop long-term wear and tear damage.

What causes misalignments?
Muscles are joined to bone by tendons and enable the body to move. Misalignments can happen when too much muscle tension causes a bone to move towards the tighter muscle. Whenever we move in an unbalanced way – for example hoovering or carrying a heavy bag on one arm – we can cause misalignments. We may also hurt ourselves through lifting, falling, childbirth, sport, or simply bad posture. Chiropractors will give you advice as to how to avoid future problems.

Benefits
Chiropractic can treat the same conditions as osteopathy, including:

• joint stiffness
• pain
• discomfort, particularly in the back, neck and shoulders
• sports injuries
• headaches and migraines

- whiplash
- sciatica
- trapped nerves and numbness.

The difference between osteopathy and chiropractic

Chiropractic and osteopathy are similar. The subtleties and developing techniques of both professions are many. It could be said that chiropractors tend to believe that manipulation is needed to put back sections of the spine that have become misaligned into the correct position, whereas osteopaths think that, although minor displacements happen, it is far more common to have the joints locking or jamming without any major displacement. Chiropractor Liz Andrews states, 'Osteopaths pull bones into place using the long levers of the body. Chiropractors push them back into place directly, using speed to overcome muscular tension. Both professions borrow techniques from each other.' Osteopath Hilary Dewey states, 'Chiropractors tend to use X-rays considerably more than osteopaths, to diagnose badly aligned joints and to suggest which way to direct their corrective thrusts. Osteopaths use X-rays mainly to exclude any serious disease, if suspected. Both professions train practitioners to consider the body as a whole. Osteopaths place more emphasis on overall posture and body mechanics while chiropractors emphasise very detailed local mechanics.'[2]

Chiropractic; the McTimoney way

This is a gentle and effective treatment for the whole body. It is a manipulative treatment that uses techniques so gentle it can be used for the very ill, the very young and the elderly. It is a very relaxing, stress-releasing therapy.

John McTimoney, a UK chiropractor in the 1950s, came to believe that the whole person should be treated, not just the problem area. He also wanted the treatment to be completely comfortable. He experimented and found that he could achieve the same results, if not better, by using very gentle techniques. He devised a whole-body chiropractic method based on what he had already been taught through Palmer's original insights and techniques. He sought to realign a patient's structure in a thorough and effective way, believing that the skull, thorax, spine, pelvis, arms and legs all have joints where bones can lose their alignment. The main technique is called the 'toggle-torque-recoil', which is performed on the vertebrae. The adjustments are precise, deft and very quick, resulting in minimum client discomfort. He started teaching this in 1972. He is believed to be the first chiropractor to have formulated a chiropractic analysis and treatment for animals.

McTimoney chiropractic aims to correct the musculo-skeletal alignment and restore nerve function to promote natural health. McTimoney practitioners do not use X-rays. If thought to be necessary to exclude disease, they would refer the patient to a doctor for X-rays. They work in cooperation with doctors wherever possible.

Rolfing

This system of bodywork is designed to change the way people relate to gravity, by systematically lengthening and repositioning the body's entire connective tissue matrix. This connective tissue, called fascia, holds the body together, both directly under the skin and on deeper levels such as around our internal organs, and groups of muscles and bones.

Like OSTEOPATHY, Rolfing seeks to enhance the body's functioning by changing its structure. However, it differs from osteopathy in that it says that repositioning the bone is not enough. Because bones are held in place by soft tissue — the muscles, ligaments, tendons and so on – if a muscle is chronically short, it will pull the bone it is attached to out of balance. The theory here is that for a change to be permanent the individual muscle and surrounding tissue must be lengthened.

Dr Ida Rolf (1896–1979), an American from New York, developed this method of deep manipulation of body structure. She was a mother, a free-thinker and a pioneer, with a single-minded desire to help others. She held a PhD in biological chemistry from the College of Physicians and Surgeons of Columbia University.

Dr Rolf asked herself what conditions must be fulfilled in order for the human body to be organised and integrated in gravity so that it can function in the most economical way. She called her system STRUCTURAL INTEGRATION and this name describes the process. Rolfing was actually a nickname, first coined at Esalen (the human growth and development centre at Big Sur, California), and has become its official name. The Rolf Institute was established in 1973 in Boulder, Colorado.

Rolfing is based on a synthesis of classical OSTEOPATHY, YOGA, and many other body practices, which Ida Rolf explored throughout the world until the end of her life. The theories of yoga influenced her in that bodies need to lengthen, and the means by which this is achieved in yoga is through taking up positions in which opposing parts of the body pull or twist each other. She believed that a balanced body gives rise to a better human being. However, to her, yoga was not enough because some contraction of the joint surfaces could not respond to the yogic positions.

The major parts of our bodies – head, shoulder, chest, hips, knees and feet – are rather like a stack of bricks. As long as the structure is correctly aligned all is well. However, our bodies can become unstable simply because of life events: physical injuries, poor posture, or emotional stress. What happens is that the connective tissue shortens and thickens in order to give extra support to wherever the troubled area is. The resulting misalignments begin in childhood and are usually long forgotten. For example, you could have had a difficult birth, such as a forceps delivery. Also children tend to copy their parents, physical mannerisms and gait. Even a minor injury such as a sprained ankle can have a long-lasting effect on the whole body, simply because of the imbalances in weight distribution that occur. Kathy Webster Bates describes the example of a sprain to the left ankle: 'Subtle changes gradually occur: the hip tilts a little to the right; the left shoulder is carried higher; and the head automatically moves to the left. Twinges of discomfort may be experienced in the lower back and or neck area.'[3]

As well as a physical structure, we are also an energy field operating in the greater energy of earth and its gravitational field. When we operate with greater structural competence we have more energy available, because we can be enhanced rather than depleted by the spatial relations of our individual energy field and that of the earth's gravitational field. In other words, when the body gets working appropriately, the force of gravity can flow through. The body can then heal itself.

Ida Rolf's method is characterised by two assumptions: firstly the radical plasticity and mobility of the bodily tissues and, secondly, the healing effects of using skilled hands to move bodily structure into alignment with the pull of gravity.

It is the concept of gravity that separates out Ida Rolf's work. Gravity is 'the omnipresent, all-powerful, unremitting determinant of their' (human beings) uprightness or lack of it. Humans are no different in their existence in gravity from any other material body. All are subject to the laws of mechanics; one of these laws states that masses must be balanced in order to be stable...'.[4]

Rolfing treatment is given over ten sessions, with each session having its own structural goals appropriate to the individual, concentrating on different parts of the body. This becomes an ongoing process of change that continues after the ten sessions. Further advanced sessions are available after a period of integration. You receive the treatment lying on a treatment couch. Photographs are taken before and after the work is completed so that changes in posture and alignment can be seen.

Ida Rolf was also associated with Fritz Perls, the grandfather of GESTALT therapy. She gave Rolfing sessions to people who were also working with Perls. Structural integration work can support psychotherapeutic work and vice versa. Areas of constricted connective tissue are indicative of chronic holding patterns that have developed because of unresolved emotional issues. When the Rolfer applies specific pressure and energy to those areas these emotions can be safely released. Ida Rolf wasn't concerned with simply 'fixing' people's pains. Clearing a pain in one part of the body meant that a new pain could appear a few days later in another place.

Benefits

Rolfing does not attempt to diagnose or cure symptoms as such. Rather it is about providing a more resilient and flexible system in which it is easier to overcome stress and ward off illness. Results vary. Here are some general benefits:

- relieves long-standing pain and fatigue brought about by poor postural habits
- enhances the performance of athletes, dancers and actors
- helps to regain a feeling of lightness and flexibility
- helps children's growing bodies develop in a balanced and coordinated way.

Contraindications

Rolfing does not claim to be a therapy for treating disease. As it is a deep pressure therapy it is best to avoid it if you are pregnant, have any infectious disease, deep vein thrombosis, shingles, painful scar tissue or varicose veins. You might want to avoid it if you bruise easily.

Postural integration

Postural integration is a development of the work of Ida Rolf by Jack Painter, an American university professor who linked ROLFING with REICHIAN THERAPY in the early seventies.

Postural integration shares with Rolfing the emphasis on the soft-tissue structure of the body. However, in addition to the relation of the body to gravity, it focuses on the inter-relatedness of the physical, emotional and thought patterns as they become evidenced in a person's posture.

The assumption is that the body stores in its cells and its patterns of muscular and energetic functioning all the past experiences of a person as well as their present feelings, thoughts, hopes and dreams. The theory is that the body is an integrated whole, a moving, thinking, feeling structure; and thus the whole person is involved in any change.

So in postural integration, the work with the soft tissues is only one aspect of the work. Attention to the thoughts and emotions that emerge during a session is seen as just as important for healing to take place. Moreover, the practitioner and the client work together and the client is very actively involved in this therapy, determining the speed and the extent of the change process at every moment. This is done both verbally and non-verbally. For example, at what level is change welcomed by the tissues of the client? Does she feel able to accept the speed and depth of touch from the therapist, or does she need it slower, or to cut off from the contact completely?

Alexander technique

'Everyone wants to be right, but no one stops to consider if their idea of right is right.' 'You can't do something you don't know if you keep on doing what you do know.' (FM Alexander).[5]

The Alexander Technique is a re-education and rediscovery, making what has been instinctive conscious through a greater awareness and understanding of how the body best functions.

Penny Ingham, Alexander teacher, says, 'Our brains tell our bodies what to do, and our bodies do as they are told. Unfortunately, during our formative years and after, most of us acquire a programme of instruction that is more or less faulty, so that our habits of posture and movement incorporate a great deal of strain and tension. It is difficult or impossible to unlearn these habits successfully; we need a means we can rely on to restore our natural poise. That means is the Alexander Technique.'

FM Alexander (1869–1955) was an actor who lost his voice at crucial moments on stage. After much careful observation he discovered that an unconscious head motion and tensing of his neck muscles interfered with his voice. He eventually cured himself and developed the Alexander Technique.

The Alexander Technique is concerned with poise rather than posture. 'Poise' conjures up images of balance, freedom of movement, lightness and fluidity. These qualities tend to be associated with young children, animals and highly trained dancers and gymnasts. In animals and young children this poise is natural. As we grow older, we lose it because we super-impose on these natural movements incorrect patterns and ways of holding ourselves, most of which are unconsciously acquired through boredom, fear, stress or imitation of our parents, heroes or peer group.

The way in which we move is unconscious and habitual. What is habitual feels right, so we can't always trust our feelings. We need to develop powers of observation of ourselves and others in order to change the way we use our bodies. The Alexander Technique is about unlearning habits of movement and posture, not by superimposing one set of habits on top of another, but by undoing patterns of tension that may be creating, for example, that stoop or stiff neck. It demands a willingness to take responsibility for the way in which we live every day in our bodies. It is more of an education than a treatment. The teacher helps you to unlearn the patterns of tension and relearn your body's ideal way of moving. You can then reduce effort and be easier with your body.

The relationship between pupil and teacher is important. At first the pupil is teacher-dependent, but soon this becomes a partnership and the learning curve is less steep. This kind of approach distinguishes the Alexander Technique from many other therapies. Usually sessions are weekly, or even more frequent, at the beginning. There are then greater intervals as the pupil becomes less teacher-dependent. The sessions usually last between thirty and forty minutes and are very gentle. You are fully clothed, except for your shoes.

Although Alexander teachers tailor sessions to pupils' individual needs, they teach within a traditional framework. They work with the movements of everyday life. As a pupil you work with your teacher, using simple positions and activities such as getting in and out of a chair or lying down. Your teacher, using her hands and voice, guides and monitors your body, both when it is still and when moving. This helps you let go of tension. Penny Ingham tells us that tension can be reworded 'doing too much'. In fact, she says, 'You can be lying on a beach and still be doing too much.'

Alexander called the relation between the head and neck the 'primary control', believing, rightly, that conditions in this area affected the functioning of the whole body. The key to new-found poise lies in the head, neck, back relationship (abbreviated to HNB). Once a correct relationship is restored between these three areas then balance and ease of movement can flow. The teaching methods include verbal instruction, demonstrations and light touch.

I remember in one of my own Alexander Technique lessons I was amazed to learn that, although I felt as if I was falling backwards, I was actually standing straight for the first time in a long time. What had become 'normal' was actually out of balance. This is one reason why a teacher is really important.

Benefits
In the Alexander Technique you acquire a more efficient and effective programme for the use of your body. So you:

- reduce back and neck tension
- reduce stress
- improve posture, appearance, mobility and consequent general well-being
- enhance performance and reduce stress in sport, the performing arts, in the workplace and in all everyday activity.

Contraindications
If you have a medical condition you may well need other treatment before receiving Alexander Technique lessons. Normally, however, provided you are taught by a fully qualified Alexander teacher, there are no dangers.

Glenda Jordan is a forty-six-year-old actress. Here is her story. (It is important to note that teachers vary in the emphasis of their lessons. Glenda's experience is unique to her and her teacher.)

'As a child I was pigeontoed – forever tripping over my feet – and had to wear foot supports, although the doctors never actually pinpointed a problem. As a teenager I began to have chronic back pain, which steadily got worse as I got older. I always knew there was something wrong with me because, when I looked in the mirror, I could see that one set of muscles beside my spine was more developed than those on the other side.

In my early twenties I tried chiropractic and osteopathic treatment, but they didn't help. In my mid twenties, I decided to try Alexander Technique, which I had heard about on the grapevine.

I remember being quite bemused by the first session. As opposed to chiropractic or osteopathy, the teacher did not manipulate my skeleton. She did look at my posture and spine, but I spent that whole session sitting down and getting up from a chair with her guiding and monitoring this with her hands. However, when I walked out on the street afterwards I had the most extraordinary experience; I felt as if I was a foot taller than everybody else. I felt euphoric, uplifted, really really high, with a tremendous sense of freedom and release.

I continued to see her for sixteen sessions, and she gave me a sort of mantra to repeat in my head: 'neck free, head rolls forward to go up, my back lengthens and widens'. Later we added: 'wide across the top of the arms and knees forward and away'.

The idea, as I understood it, was to re-educate the musculature of the head, neck and back so that the weight of the upper part of the body no longer compressed the spine. I did this by thinking about my body and releasing the muscles (not by sitting up straight, which actually makes the spine shorter, putting you off balance). As well as sitting down and standing up, my teacher worked with me in other ordinary situations, like walking, standing, lying down. All the time I would be thinking of lengthening and widening and thinking against my habit of pulling down. This is a fine example of the connection between body and mind for me.

At the end of the sessions I was, I swear to God, half an inch taller than when I started. By rebalancing my body, the space between the vertebrae had increased.

I don't consider the Alexander Technique a cure because it didn't straighten my pelvis, but perhaps if I'd had more sessions this would have improved. However, what it did provide me with is the long-term successful management of the situation. I know, for instance, if I hoover by bending from the waist rather than using my knees and bending from the hips, I will get back pain. In fact, I have not had chronic back pain since my sessions, and that's twenty years ago.

I would highly recommend Alexander Technique, particularly individual classes, as they pinpoint a situation and work towards a resolution much more quickly and accurately.'

Self-help

Poised relaxation in semi-supine: this is an Alexander Technique self-help exercise. I am grateful to Penny Ingham for contributing the written notes that she gives to her pupils when working with them.

In the Alexander Technique you lie down to do work. As a mechanical fact the discs in one's spine after four or five hours of being upright need to re-absorb spinal fluid to stay healthily functional (think of it like petrol in the car). This process takes around fifteen minutes and only happens if the spine is horizontal. Lying down will also encourage the gentle curvature of your spine to re-establish, especially as you enhance this process by giving yourself directions and thinking of lengthening and widening.

Find time to work in semi-supine after five or so hours of being vertical; ie around twice a day. You need a warm carpeted room, a pile of slim paperback books and around twenty minutes (although if you've only time for five minutes, that is still beneficial).

Lie down on your back with your head resting on the books and your knees drawn up and pointing towards the ceiling. Your head should be supported by the books on the lower, flatter part of your head and with your neck clear. The height of the books is to establish what Alexander called HNB (head, neck, back) alignment. With too few books your chin will stick up towards the ceiling and with too many your chin will push down into your throat. The books should support your head in such as way that it rolls slightly towards your chest, does not pull back, and allows your neck to lengthen.

Let your elbows rest on the floor as far out to the side as possible, with your hands palm down, resting on your body. Let your wrists soften and drop and your fingers spread.

Place your feet about one foot's length away from your bottom, with the inside of your feet on a line along from the outside of your hips (so you are in a deep, fairly wide lying down 'squat'). Your knees point to the ceiling, but your kneecaps drop down and out towards your little toes. This is a description of your legs when they are balancing with minimum effort. (If your legs were tense, your knees would pull together.) Let your ankles relax so that your knees drift outwards with the soles of your feet still in contact with the floor. Think of the under-surface of your feet. If your legs are really balanced, the weight will distribute around the outside of your feet like a perfect footprint but *not* down on the arch.

Think of your back lengthening and widening as you give your directions. Your spine will gradually realign itself quite naturally. Its natural curves will be re-establishing; you will start to feel more contact with the floor and the discs in your spine will be re-absorbing fluid, so restoring their size, shape and resilience.

Now the whole of your spine can settle. Feel the floor and the books supporting you. You are making friends with gravity!

Chapter Seven
Zones, Meridians and Pressure Point Therapies

These therapies are generally based on theories that originally come from the Far East, including countries such as China, Japan and Korea. There are energy lines or pathways called meridians that flow inside the body and extend outside the body. These pathways each have a direction of energy flow and this can be activated by precise touch on particular points on the body. Zones refer to a system of dividing up the body into ten segments or channels running vertically through the body and ending in the feet and hands. Although based on a similar concept that accurate pressure on one point (called a reflex point) on the body affects related organs or areas in other parts of the body, these zones are not the same as meridians. Zone therapy has a different historical and cultural background; it is much more recent, having originated in Connecticut, America in the early 1900s (see REFLEXOLOGY, which developed out of Zone therapy).

Treatments using zones, meridians and pressure points do not separate out physical symptoms from the movement or stagnation of the energy that flows through the body. I have included ACUPUNCTURE here because it involves direct contact with the body, albeit through very fine needles. The theories and ancient tradition of acupuncture inform many of the more modern bodywork therapies, eg TOUCH FOR HEALTH and POLARITY THERAPY, now available in the West.

Chinese medicine

Chinese medicine is a vast historical tradition that has never been merely one institution. Over the millennia a great many doctors have developed its theories and techniques and, as it develops in different countries, it adapts to these cultures and ever-changing social demands.

However, fundamentally, traditional Chinese philosophy tells us that our health is dependent on the body's motivating energy – chi – moving in a smooth and balanced way through a series of channels, called meridians, beneath our skin. Chi (sometimes spelt 'ki' or 'qi' and pronounced *chee*) consists of equal and opposite qualities, yin and yang. When these become unbalanced, illness may result. Upset in the smooth flow of chi causes blockages or dams in some areas, and weakness or stagnant pools in others. This may lead to serious illness, or simply to a feeling that 'things are just not quite right'. This flow of chi can be disturbed by many factors, including poor nutrition, anxiety, stress, weather conditions, hereditary factors, infections, poisons and general physical and emotional traumas.

Yin and yang are two concepts fundamental to Chinese philosophy. Yin represents the female energy and yang the male. These energies aren't about gender as such, but rather are about polar opposites, or complements. Within yin and yang is the possibility of opposite and change. Harmony between these elements brings optimum health; imbalance results in disease. Yin qualities include inwardness, downwardness, cold, winter, emotion, passivity, darkness, softness and the moon. Yang qualities include outwardness, upwardness, heat, summer, assertion, activity, hardness, verbal and logic, and the sun. Illnesses are categorised as yin or yang. For example, hot, over-active, forceful symptoms are yang, and weakness, slowness, coldness and underactivity are yin. Yin and yang define one another – you cannot have light without knowing dark – and they control and balance each other.

Out of a complex medical system, only the bare essentials of technique have reached the West, although recently authentic Chinese clinics from China are opening in the UK to respond to public interest. The full clinical potential and theoretical depth of Chinese medicine remain virtually unknown. Based on ancient texts, it is the result of a continuous process of critical thinking, as well as extensive clinical observation and testing by respected physicians. As Ted Kaptchuk states: 'It is also, however, rooted in the philosophy, logic, sensibility and habits of a civilisation entirely foreign to our own.'[1] He uses an excellent example to describe the difference between Chinese and Western medicine: when a Western physician is confronted by a patient who has stomach pain, he or she must look beyond the screen of symptoms for an underlying pathological mechanism, such as a peptic ulcer, infection, tumour or nervous disorder. The Chinese physician examining the same patient would need to discern a pattern of disharmony made up of an entire accumulation of symptoms and signs. From the Western viewpoint the Chinese physician is assessing the patient's specific and general physiological and psychological response to a disease entity.

Traditional Chinese medicine found its way into Europe centuries ago – a herbal text written in 1587 came into the hands of German physicians in 1605. As Chinese immigrants came to the US in the mid-1800s, their medicine came with them. At around the same time, the Chinese were learning the value of Western medical practices; that in certain life-threatening situations, Western medical and surgical techniques can be most appropriate. Either system can be chosen for functional disorders. However, Western medicine has considerable limitations on what it can offer to help chronic degenerative disorders, whereas traditional Chinese medicine offers more. In China sometimes both systems are used. For example, cancer sufferers may have surgery, radiation or chemotherapy and use traditional medicine for strengthening the body and immunity. Patients can then tolerate the Western treatment more easily.

Traditional Chinese medicine consists of many different aspects, including acupuncture, herbs, diet, massage, meditation, exercising and moxibustion (applying heat through the burning of a herb called moxa, which stimulates chi energy at acupuncture points). In China applying pressure on points on the body is usually an important part of massage techniques and is called Tui-na. In Japan massage techniques are called SHIATSU. Shiatsu also includes pressure of points, working along the whole length of meridians using thumbs, heels of the hand and even feet. It also includes manipulation and stretching of limbs.

Because Chinese culture has been concerned with the state, the collective and the family – not the individual – Chinese psychology is wrapped up in these systems. We are each an ecosystem and we live within one. As Beinfeld and Korngold state, '... because Chinese medical theory assumes human process unfolds as a consequence of the tension and unity between interacting systems, mental phenomena are not considered to be altogether separate or distinct from physical events.' They also go on to say, 'Because our perception of the world influences how we live in it, our consciousness sculpts reality. Conversely, our experience shapes our thinking, so our reality moulds consciousness. Our minds create what is real, and our lived experiences generate our thoughts. There is a reciprocity between beliefs and observations...'.[2] So how we make sense of our bodies will depend on what our beliefs are.

Prevention is a key focus: 'Maintaining order rather than correcting disorder is the ultimate principle of wisdom. To cure disease after it has appeared is like digging a well when one already feels thirst, or forging weapons after the war has already begun.'[3] This is not to say that we won't or shouldn't get ill sometimes, rather that we can manage it when we do and can accumulate resources when we are well. So how we manage our vital energy and balance rest, activity, food and so on is essential. In this system there is not a search for a single remedy, a magic pill, but rather the doctor and patient engaging in an ongoing process of learning what is needed to get well.

The human body is viewed as a garden; a dynamic self-regulating system that transforms water (yin) and sunlight (yang) into living vegetation within natural seasonal cycles. Plants need the best growing conditions so that they can be resilient. They need to be tended, growth promoted in some areas, restricted in others, the soil kept fertile, watered in times of drought and so on. This is the same with the human body. It is also subject to the rhythms and cycles of nature.

Exploring Chinese medicine can be very confusing. For instance there are two usages of the term traditional Chinese medicine. It originally referred to the many different schools of thought that developed over thousands of years in China. However at the time of the cultural revolution in the 1960s, there was a desire to standardise medicine. What was then taken and called traditional Chinese medicine was actually 'the eight principles approach', which has been predominantly used in Chinese herbal medicine. The eight principles are made up of four pairs of opposites; yin/yang, interior/exterior, deficiency/excess and cold/hot. Because of the totality of the nature of the yin/yang relationship, it is the dominant force in these eight principles.

The Five Element approach, which is also practised in the West, was one of the many approaches in existence before the cultural revolution. The diagnosing is based on the relationships between the five basic elements of the universe: fire, water, metal, wood and earth. In Japan the Five Element system has persisted as a very strong influence and has a great emphasis on palpating the 'hara' in order to make a diagnosis. The hara is the name given to the area around the abdomen from the pubic bone up to the rib cage and palpation involves gentle or deep probing pressure with the fingers.

Acupuncture

Acupuncture is one aspect of Chinese medicine. It offers us a totally different way of treatment from conventional Western medicine, using different concepts and methods of diagnosis. For example, the pulse is taken in six different positions in each wrist to feel for the quality and strength rather than just the speed.

Benefits

Many people who choose acupuncture have a huge range of conditions, such as:

- anxiety states
- back pain
- circulatory problems
- asthma
- arthritis
- depression
- general aches and pains
- infertility
- menstrual problems
- migraines
- skin conditions or ulcers.

It is important to note that acupuncture can be used for emotional and mental illnesses, as well as physical ones. There is really nothing that acupuncture cannot treat. It can help significantly during pregnancy and has been proved to be of help in relieving pain during childbirth. It can also help overcome addictions to smoking, alcohol, food or drugs. It can help to regulate irregular heart function, correct blood pressure, and help the production of red and white blood cells. The benefits are often more than just relief from a particular condition. You may find that you have increased energy, a better appetite and sleep, as well as having an overall improvement in your sense of well-being. You can have acupuncture as a preventive measure to strengthen your constitution and it can also be used along with conventional medicine for both chronic and acute conditions.

Conventional Western doctors see acupuncture as limited to pain relief. Neurophysiological experiments have shown that acupuncture modifies the transmission of neural (nerve) impulses between the spinal cord and the brain. This is called 'gate control' theory, which postulates that acupuncture blocks the action of pain fibres in the spinal cord by stimulating the release of endorphins (brain hormones that the body produces in response to stress). These endorphins give us a sense of euphoria. However, this hypothesis does not explain the diverse therapeutic effects of acupuncture.

There are about five hundred recognised acupuncture points on the body and about one hundred of these are commonly used. Stimulation of specific areas on the skin affects the functioning of certain organs in the body. However, those areas may not be close to the part of the body where the problem is felt. For example, you may be suffering from headaches, but needles may be inserted in your hand or your foot.

The patient's disharmonies are diagnosed in terms of excesses or deficiencies of yin and yang energy and the meridian systems most intimately related to the disharmony are identified. Acupuncture may help the flow of chi by strengthening it or helping it to flow better if there is stagnation.

The skills that the acupuncturist draws on in making her diagnosis include looking, hearing, smelling, questioning and touching; she may observe your tongue, or listen to the sound of your breathing. Specific questions are asked to ascertain signs of excess/deficiency, heat/cold, interior/exterior and yin/yang, and to gain relevant information about your history and background. Through palpation of the hara the practitioner will look for any areas of discomfort, tenderness, or blocked energy (chi).

Sensing the flow of chi through touch is a high art, the subtleties of which take many years to learn. The practitioner feels what is happening in a specific area, such as tightness, hardness or flaccidity. The abdomen is prone to imbalance, common causes being poor diet or digestion, or through energetic blocks caused by emotional turmoil. Certain areas of the hara relate to specific meridians. There can be particular tender points on the hara, which some schools of acupuncture refer to as 'alarm points'. These points will indicate specific problem areas.

The acupuncturist feels your pulse in six places on the radial artery of both wrists. Each position corresponds to a meridian. These meridians are areas of high chi concentration. The distribution of chi is a very complex system. Needles are inserted at certain access points along these meridians, and may be withdrawn immediately or retained for twenty to thirty minutes. Acupuncture needles are not like the ones we are used to when we receive injections or blood tests; they are much finer and are solid rather than hollow. Neither are they like sewing needles or pins. They are very fine, more like a hair.

Concerns about HIV have led to most practitioners using disposable needles, which are only used once. Any registered practitioner follows strict sterile procedures, whether needles are disposable or not.

Dianne Summers, traditional acupuncturist, tells us, 'In the West few people realise the full depth and beauty of Chinese medicine. For example, every classical point has a name: Greater Mountain Stream, Heavenly Spring, Blazing Valley, Spirit Path, Soul Door and so on. Every point is at a precise anatomical location, and needle depth varies as does manipulation of the needle. Training to do traditional practice is extensive both in Chinese medicine and Western orthodox medicine. To practise is an art; perhaps this contributes to the difficulties scientists experience. For here both the objective and subjective approaches need to come together. So research goes on, but that which has stood the test of time must surely be saying something and results more than mere imagining.'

What are you likely to feel?

The most common sensations felt when a needle is inserted is a dull ache or tingling, not a pinprick. Depending on what therapeutic aim the practitioner has she may move the needle by lightly twisting or manipulating it.

Number and frequency of treatments will vary according to the problem. Typically you may need weekly sessions for ten to fifteen weeks, but some people only need one or two. Where there is chronic illness, or people are choosing to maintain or seek optimum health, they may have treatment for several years.

As with all the therapies, theory and practice within Chinese medicine, and acupuncture in particular, are developing all the time. New names you may come across are TRIGGER POINT or MYOFASCIAL ACUPUNCTURE and AURICULAR ACUPUNCTURE. The former refer to the work of Mark Seem in the US, in which the myofascial layers of tissue in specific energetic zones of the body are worked on using acupuncture, creating balance at a much more systemic – that is, deeper – level in the body (4). The latter refers to the identification of the whole body in the ear (the ear is like a map representing all the parts of the body) and special needles are used. There is also ELECTRO-ACUPUNCTURE – the use of a small DC electric current between pairs of needles – which is primarily for pain relief.

Contraindications

Acupuncture can be harmful if used incorrectly. You must see a fully qualified practitioner. She or he should advise you as to what treatment is appropriate and will monitor your responses very carefully.

Mary is English, and in her mid-forties. She is a social historian, a writer, and is training to be a healer herself. She writes about her experiences of acupuncture:

'For me, acupuncture has worked and continues to help me to shift energy blocks and work with stagnant energy – it is always a release. Having an acupuncture treatment is like a meditation; going into a dreamlike place and finding my body enveloped in a sea of healing energy.

Like most therapies it's not a quick fix. One has to be patient and work with it gradually. I have integrated it into my life as an aid to well-being, rather than a therapy I use when I'm ill. That said, I have experienced a couple of 'quick fixes'. For many years I had a sebaceous cyst[5] on my head. Once when I was staying in New York it started getting bigger and was painful, so I went to see a wonderful old Chinese man (a doctor trained in both traditions, as is the way in China) in China Town. In a few minutes, with tongue and pulse diagnosis, he prescribed me a batch of herbs, all wrapped in neatly folded envelopes of paper and to be boiled and drunk. Within three days the cyst had disappeared and has never returned!

Acupuncture works on the level of energy; I feel as though the whole of me is central to the healing process. It doesn't involve a lot of discussion. I generally say how I feel and the diagnosis is tongue and pulse. My feeling is that the strongest treatments are given by Chinese practitioners, ie Chinese or Western practitioners who trained in China. Yes, it can be painful but only momentarily (when the needle hits the energy block), not once the needles are in place. It helps if one has an awareness of diet/exercise, lifestyle and stress issues, so that these can be worked on alongside the treatments.'

Here is the story of Lorraine, a middle-aged woman who followed up conventional treatment for cancer with acupuncture:

'Late in 1989 I was feeling generally unwell and, on recommendation of friends, went to an acupuncturist...In 1990 I was diagnosed as having cancer of the bladder. This was dealt with in the early stages by laser operation and, while it is not a particularly threatening form of cancer, I decided that it would be a good idea to continue with acupuncture as a means of keeping myself in balance. While I was recovering from the operation (and the shock), I went every fortnight but my acupuncturist advised me when it was time for less frequent visits.

I now go once a month. It keeps me in balance. It also helps my arthritis. Overwork is a character trait (although I have become a little more sensible) and it is good for me not only physically but because my acupuncturist, although not saying much about my lifestyle, is a constant reminder to me that I should be more careful. We talk about books, films, politics, religion, the garden. Also, through our discussions over the years and her sensitive and professional approach, I have come to understand that I am capable of reading my own body and its symptoms to a certain extent. This means that I am more likely to keep an eye on my excesses of work. There are times when she has to put needles into the sides of my feet or my toes, which can be painful, but the pain is so transient as not to matter. I often feel sleepy a short while after a visit, but always feel better for it.'

Shiatsu

As with ACUPUNCTURE, shiatsu involves connecting with energy channels (meridians) and specific points on the body. It is a hands-on therapy, sometimes described as 'acupuncture without the needles'. Practitioners work with diagnosing in the same way as acupuncturists; balancing the chi, and clearing blockages in energy. Literally translated, shiatsu means 'finger pressure'.

CHINESE MEDICINE was brought to Japan about one thousand years ago. About one hundred years ago, European medicine was introduced to Japan and adopted by the aristocracy. This affected the continuation of native healing methods and the practise of massage techniques was disallowed. However, during the 1920s the first law to regulate ancient therapies was introduced in Japan, and in 1925 the Shiatsu Therapists Association was created. In Japan shiatsu has developed into a major healing art and practitioners are regarded as experts in treating many ailments. It is offered for free as a health-care method to workers in major industry, and most Japanese families will know how to use simple shiatsu massage techniques in the home.

In shiatsu a wide range of hand techniques are used. Pressure is applied using the thumbs, fingers, palms, elbows, forearms and sometimes the feet to meridians, or to a specific point, called a tsubo. The practitioner may also use stretches to initiate the movement of chi in the meridians. Joints may be put through their range of motion in order to increase flexibility. Treatment follows a set pattern, which is likely to vary according to which school of shiatsu the practitioner trained at. The practitioner uses a form of diagnosis by touching (palpating) your back and abdomen (the hara). Like the acupuncturist, the shiatsu practitioner uses various forms of diagnosis to assess the amount of chi in the meridians. She endeavours to find a link between cause and effect on all levels of the person's being so that the underlying causes of the problems are uncovered. During the session you are worked on with your clothes on. These need to be loose and comfortable, and you will be lying down on a padded mat or futon on the floor.

Benefits

Shiatsu works on many chronic conditions such as:

- back pain
- migraine
- arthritis
- asthma
- insomnia
- sciatica
- constipation.

Shiatsu is used during pregnancy and, like REFLEXOLOGY, can be used very specifically for gynaecological and general health problems. It is particularly helpful in preventing and countering stress-related disorders, helping to build resistance to frequent colds, flu and general aches and pains.

Shiatsu practitioner Jill Carter tells us: 'This deeply relaxing bodywork aims to bring all the elements of our nature back to balance, but the very effort of living is sometimes about disharmony and distress. For some women, then, the sessions are simply an oasis of peace, just an hour for themselves. For another individual it is a positive way to address and heal a tendency towards painful periods, perhaps experienced since puberty. For the young mother raw with the grief of losing her baby there can be some solace and easing of the ache her womb feels through receiving gentle ampuku (massage) to the belly. Then there can be the career woman who comes regularly for sessions to develop confidence. Yet another laughs with delight on being advised to gather rose petals and float them in her bath to celebrate being a woman.'

When you receive shiatsu you will find that each session is very different. The form is highly creative. Sometimes it is dynamic with pressure, kneading and stretching, and at other times it seems as if nothing much is happening, when in fact the practitioner is holding or warmly cupping areas of depletion. Shiatsu works well with traditional Chinese herbal and dietary medicine, and practitioners generally give specific advice on diet and lifestyle.

Practitioners are trained to recognise symptoms that require conventional Western medical attention and will encourage the patient to see her GP if necessary. *Shiatsu for Women* by Ray Ridolfe and Susanne Franzen is an excellent resource book, especially on self-help techniques (see Selected Reading).

One partial Western explanation for the beneficial effects of shiatsu is that, by stimulating pressure points, it is able to diffuse the lactic acid and carbon monoxide that accumulates in muscle tissue, causing stiffness and sluggishness in the blood flow, which puts pressure on the nerves, the blood and lymph vessels. This then affects the bones and internal organs. Clearing blockages in points means the energy along the meridians is able to flow clearly.

Ridolfe and Susanne Franzen state: 'Women particularly seem to be attracted to shiatsu. Many more women than men come for treatments and the majority of those studying shiatsu as a career are also women. We think that this may be because women tend to be more aware of their own bodies and the concept of feeling good about themselves, whereas men perhaps are more inclined to ignore signs and symptoms of imbalance until much later.'[6] They go on to say that we could see the menstrual cycle as an advantage because when there are unexpected changes we cannot help but be aware of them.

There are other forms of shiatsu that you may come across, which are developments from general shiatsu practice. These include TANTSU, which focuses on the chakra system; MACRO-BIOTIC SHIATSU, which includes dietary guidance and medicinal plant foods as well as hands-on touch and pressure; and BAREFOOT SHIATSU, which employs the fingers, palms and feet of the practitioner, and is a component of macrobiotic shiatsu.

Shiatsu can be used alongside other forms of treatment that strengthen the constitution or support the person's develop-ment and well-being. Although technically not real shiatsu, some massage practitioners use shiatsu techniques or concepts as part of their massage, or incorporate these into an AROMATHERAPY session, usually following a set pattern of points to either relax or revitalise. Someone trained in Chinese medicine may also take your pulses (as in acupuncture) and they may diagnose your tongue.

Contraindications

Certain points are not used in early pregnancy because of possible risk of miscarriage. With a well-trained practitioner there is no danger, as they know which points to avoid.

Other contraindications are if you:

- have a high fever
- are intoxicated
- have just eaten (a treatment should be given two hours or more after meals)

- have chronic high blood pressure (medical advice should be sought)
- have a history of brain haemorrhage
- have blood-borne cancer
- have a skin or air 'contact' contagious disease.

As with other therapies, you should not be treated if you have had recent surgery. The practitioner should not put pressure over varicose veins, or use deep pressure during a period. If you are an HIV/AIDS sufferer it is safe, because no body fluids are exchanged.

Acupressure

Acupressure theory is also based on the precepts of CHINESE MEDICINE. It is much more point focused than shiatsu. It involves the stimulation of specific points (acupuncture points) along the meridians, using thumb, finger or knuckle pressure, or a blunt instrument called a tei shin (a wooden knob with a rounded tip).

Pressure points are located by referring to anatomy, such as how close they are to bone. They have Chinese names that describe their nature. For example, Spleen 10 which helps release suppressed menses is called 'Ocean of blood'. Techniques involve pressing (dian qia), pinching (nie na), pushing and rolling, friction (gua sha liao fa), rubbing and stretching strokes.

Tui–na is an ancient system of massage/bodywork based on Chinese medicine, which here is classified under acupressure. Tui–na can also include bone setting, ie orthopaedic manipulations. References to Tui–na were made as early as 300 BC and by AD 591 a department of massage had been established at the Imperial College of Medicine in China. 'Tui' means to push and 'na' to grasp.

Today this treatment is taught in all traditional medical schools in the People's Republic of China. There are a number of different styles and specific manipulations within Tui-na and these came down from different lineages or traditions. Tui-na is sometimes gentle but sometimes vigorous. Different methods of exerting pressure on points often involve a lot of repetition.

Several major schools of Chinese therapeutic massage are recognised within Tui-na. One of these is called the 'one-finger school', in which one finger is used to stimulate acupuncture points along the meridians, the force being concentrated through the tip of the thumb. This system is deemed effective in the treatment of gynaecological problems. Another is the 'rolling school', which came out of the one-finger school. This method covers larger body surfaces.

Benefits
Tui-na is used to treat many conditions. Here are just a few:

- headaches
- high blood pressure
- menstrual problems
- asthma
- arthritis
- sore throats
- sinus congestion
- back and neck pain
- hayfever.

Another widely available form of acupressure is called **Jin Shin Do**. This derives partially from an art called 'Jin hin jitus', which is based on traditional Japanese acupressure methods, as well as meditation techniques. Gentle, yet firm, direct finger or thumb pressure on acupressure points may sound simple, but this form of touch is capable of infinite development in its subtleties.

In order to release trapped chi energy the amount of pressure needs to be right, not too light or too heavy. Practitioners use a complex system of working with pressure points and meridians.

To work with the whole person, Jin Shin Do practitioners use breathing, meditation, exercise methods and traditional dietary principles to keep the body-mind in balance. The method emphasises developing and maintaining well-being, rather than concentrating on a symptomatic approach. It aims at a deep release and rejuvenation, through which the higher, or psychic, centres can be opened.

Contraindications

Do not receive acupressure if:

- you have an acute infection
- you have recently eaten
- you have exercised strenuously
- you have a skin disease, ulcerations or inflammations near a point.

There are a lot of overlaps between these Chinese and Japanese styles of acupressure. They are all variations on a theme of traditional oriental medicine, but using somewhat different methods of treating and balancing chi.

Reflexology

Reflexology is another ancient technique of treating the whole body by pressing reflex points in the foot or hand. It was being used over five thousand years ago in India and China. It possibly goes back further to ancient Egypt. Pictographs found in the tomb of an Egyptian physician 2500–2300 BC show a man being given a form of reflexology.

It has also been found to exist in many African tribes and Native Americans, especially the Cherokee people.

Pressure may either be applied to points that are directly involved with a particular condition or to points that are associated. These are called direct reflexes or associated reflexes.

It can also help with sleep patterns, relaxation and well-being. Reflexology is both a treatment and a diagnostic tool. A skilled reflexologist can tell you your medical history and current problems by feeling your feet. Legally, however, reflexologists are not allowed to diagnose medically.

In 1983 in Germany a Dr Alfons Cornelius found that having regular massage with an emphasis on the painful spots meant he recovered from infection. However, it was Dr William Fitzgerald, an American ear, nose and throat specialist, who popularised a new therapy called ZONE THERAPY in 1902. Fitzgerald divided the body into ten zones. Energy flowing throughout each zone links all the areas of the body situated in the same zone. The same zones exist in both the legs and arms and this means that parts of the body are 'zone related' on the same side. Related zones are the shoulder and hip, the upper arm and upper leg, the elbow and knee, the forearm and the lower leg, the wrist and the ankle and the hand and foot (the palm of the hand relating to the sole of the foot and the back of the hand relating to the top of the foot). There are also four zones going across the body that relate to the levels of the shoulder girdle, diaphragm, waist and pelvic floor. Reflex points run throughout and any tension or blockage in any part of the zone will affect the whole zone, just as direct pressure on any part of the zone will also affect the whole zone.

Another American, Eunice Ingham, developed zone therapy into reflexology by concentrating on reflex points on the feet and hands.

Different areas of the feet were found to correspond to different body systems eg big toe – head and brain; rest of toes – the sinuses; lungs spread across the ball of the foot and the lower back down in the heel. The reflexology technique loosens tensions and relieves blockages in the flow of energy to the corresponding body part of the system.

Her pupil Doreen Bailey brought reflexology to the UK in 1966. Now reflexology has gained respectability and is used in some GP surgeries, hospitals and hospices.

Benefits

The benefits of reflexology treatment are wide and include help with:

- alleviating pain
- improving blood circulation
- the functioning of the eliminatory systems (clearing unwanted toxins from the body)
- menstrual problems, such as amenorrhoea (absence of periods), dysmenorrhoea (painful periods) and metrorrhagia (irregular periods)
- PMS
- infertility
- unpleasant symptoms during pregnancy, such as sickness and nausea, constipation, backache, sciatica and increased frequency of passing urine
- postnatal symptoms including tiredness, depression, urinary infections, breast discomfort, depression, insomnia, headaches, failing memory, indigestion, flatulence, constipation, increased frequency of passing urine, thinning of skin, atrophy of the breasts, mastitis (inflammation of the breasts), loss of interest in sex, hot flushes and osteoporosis (brittle bones)
- inflammatory conditions such as endometriosis (endometrium tissues found in abnormal sites in the body, often the ovaries, fallopian tubes and pelvic structures) and vaginitis (inflammation of the vagina).

These conditions, especially if chronic, need to be taken seriously and your medical doctor needs to know about them. As reflexology has gained a fair degree of acceptance within the medical profession, hopefully your doctor would support you if you chose to seek help with reflexology.

Reflexologist Nicola Hall says, 'Many midwives now use reflexology to help at the time of childbirth, particularly to help with pain or if birth is delayed or uterine contractions are weak.'[8]

Sometimes the menstrual cycle alters temporarily during or after a course of reflexology; periods may come slightly earlier or be slightly heavier. This shouldn't last long. As regards an intrauterine device, or IUD, Nicola Hall states, '. . . in some instances this may be detected during reflexology treatment as being a "foreign" item in the body and the device, particularly if it is not fitted well, may move. Although this is not a common reaction, it is one to be aware of.'[9]

Contraindications

Reflexology can be painful, especially if you are sensitive. A good practitioner will always check if the pressure is okay for you.

Reflexology should not be given if you:

- have an infectious disease
- have a fever or very high temperature
- have deep vein thrombosis
- have just had replacement surgery
- suffer with severe osteoporosis, the decalcification of the bones, especially in the feet and hands
- are experiencing an unstable pregnancy.

In addition extra care needs to be given if you have a heart condition, are pregnant, epileptic, diabetic or are on medication. If you are taking painkillers, tranquillisers or antidepressants, this can sometimes numb the reflexes. Too much pressure could inadvertently be applied because you may not feel, or therefore report, any tenderness. However, the effects are still taking place.

Beware, also, of using reflexology, feeling better, and having a deeper condition masked. Jill is in her fifties now and is a very busy social worker. Here is her experience:

'In 1980 my father-in-law died rather suddenly and, a few weeks later, my own father died from a heart attack. In between the two deaths, I was taken ill myself but was told by my GP that it was "trauma". I didn't think so for various reasons but could not convince him otherwise so went to consult the naturopath I had been seeing. She did not know what it was either but felt that it was somehow linked to my womb and asked me to go back to my GP.

The naturopath was also a reflexologist and she gave me a reflexology treatment. I had never heard of it before and, as well as having all the other pains I was suffering from at the time, I ended up with a sore foot, which I could barely put to the ground! However, the following day, I realised that both the pain in my foot and the other pains had gone, which was quite amazing. In retrospect, I now think this could have been somewhat dangerous as it became even more difficult to convince my GP that there was anything the matter with me. But eventually I did and it turned out that I had had an ectopic pregnancy, which necessitated surgery.'

Here is Carole Wood's experience of reflexology. She sent it to me in diary form:

'Within a three-year period I had experienced more negative life events than I was able to cope with: the loss of a business and, with it, the loss of a long and valued friendship with business partners. This resulted in the loss of my home. Furniture was sold to buy food. My daughter was uprooted from the friends and neighbours she had grown to love. My husband was unable to cope with the pressure and turned in on himself. We had moved to a damp, old mill house, a stop-gap until we could be rehoused, as lodgers.

Following all this my mother discovered that she had cancer of the womb. The day I was to accompany her to Christies in Manchester for intensive treatment, I myself was rushed into hospital suffering an ectopic pregnancy that almost claimed my life.

I had no reserves with which to fight back. I knew that I could go down the route of antidepressant drugs to help me to cope or that I could try the 'alternative' route and lift my depression and utter exhaustion with the help of complementary therapies.

I decided on a course of reflexology from a practitioner I knew well and trusted. She came to my home to treat me. I combined this treatment with meditation and a healthy meat-free diet, rich in vitamins and minerals. The following is an account taken from diaries at the time:

Session one: Feel down in the dumps today and almost rang to cancel my reflexology session. I cannot see any light in the world. We all have a flu bug, exacerbated by this awful damp house. My feet are extremely sensitive. O worked very gently over the areas corresponding to the chest and sinuses. My blocked-up nose actually started running during the treatment! I found the area corresponding to the womb, etc, very tender, but so soon after surgery this was to be expected. O's touch had been very light and gentle.

Felt much better after O's visit. In fact I fell asleep in the chair for an hour. A blessed relief from the awful dark depression that has beset me. If only the beneficial effects of the treatment could have lasted longer. Went to bed happier but again could not sleep.

Session two: The flu symptoms seem to be receding, though I am left with a dreadful cough. O concentrated on the area corresponding to the lungs and bronchial tubes and also, of course, on the area corresponding to the womb, which is still very tender. I feel a little better today, rested after the treatment and put on some music and gave myself a guided meditation. I am sure that if I can only hold hope and beauty in my heart then I can get through this. Sleeping a little better, at least no nightmares for four days.

Session three: The flu seems to have gone and I feel physically better and more alive. Enjoyed the session with O but made the mistake of rushing down to the mill to help Brian. Felt tired out tonight and quite spaced out; I must organise the session so that I have time to rest afterwards and allow the healing to sink in.

Session four: A beautiful session today. O says she can see and feel an improvement in the colour and texture of the skin on my feet. Was overwhelmed with emotion after O's visit. Grieved over all aspects of mothering; grieved for my mother going through horrendous cancer treatment with the help of my father but without me to hold her hand. Grieved for myself, for the happy, stable life I felt I had deprived my daughter of, and for the loss of a brother or sister for her that she would have so loved. I kept seeing visions of a beautiful baby boy, now safe in the spirit world. I so longed to hold him in my arms and can only hold him in my heart.

Sleeping better and felt better to cry it all out. I feel drained and yet I feel at peace for the first time in three years.

Session five: I feel I can just lie back and enjoy the treatment in a state of meditation. I do have a little more energy and no longer spend my days staring at the walls. I think O sees an improvement in me and I bless her for being such an important part of my healing.

Session six: I continue to improve. This is O's last session with me, but I have been working on my feet myself and am continuing to feel the benefit. I know I have a long way to go but I feel an important start has been made on the long haul back to full health. The sun is peeping from behind the clouds!'

I find this account very moving. It highlights the gradual nature of the healing process and the oneness of body and mind.

Polarity therapy

Polarity therapy is another way of stimulating and harmonising the flow of this vital energy we call chi, or prana. This energy comes into us through air, food, light and heat, physical touch, and experiencing spirituality and love.

Polarity therapy was developed by Dr Randolph Stone (1890–1981), an Austrian who emigrated to the US when he was a young teenager. He initially studied CHIROPRACTIC, OSTEOPATHY and NATUROPATHY. Polarity therapy reflects his multidisciplinary approach, especially as he spent his life researching and studying different systems such as CHINESE MEDICINE and ACUPUNCTURE, AYURVEDIC MEDICINE and YOGA.

Dr Stone worked regularly in India, providing a free clinic for the destitute, which he considered a fair test for the effectiveness of this therapy. He believed the life force in humans is precisely the same as the life force in the whole of creation. 'It whirls round in the smallest microscopic cell in the same manner that it spins in the largest galaxy.'[10] He taught that all living things have a positive, negative and neutral pole and that energy flows from the centre of any system to its circumference and returns by magnetic pull. He believed it flows from the top downwards, and from within to without. He also used the Indian concept of chakras (see Chapter 8). In polarity therapy these chakras, or energy centres, are places where the three currents – pingala (positively charged), ida (negatively charged) and susumna (vertical neutral current) – cross over. Each chakra is governed by a particular element: earth, water, fire, air or ether.

Polarity therapy is based on the premise that we and everything else are made up of these five elements. These in turn are governed by the opposing and complementary forces of yin and yang and govern different aspects of our being:

- water: pleasure and sexuality
- fire: the will and personal power
- earth: survival and the material world
- air: movement and mental activity
- ether: creativity and personal self-expression.

If we are out of balance in any of these areas we will not be functioning well. For example too little or too much in:

- water could mean we become overwhelmed by our emotions
- fire could mean over aggressiveness, a bitter taste in the mouth, or a lack of vitality
- earth could mean we are too rigid about our routines and lack vision
- air could make us restless, anxious, stuck in old thought patterns
- ether means we could be 'off the planet', unable to manifest anything in material form.

Rosamund Webster describes the aim of this therapy: 'The practitioner works to rebalance the whole person by looking at the polarity relationship within the body (positive, negative and neutral) while working the various reflex and pressure points.'[11]

Because this therapy is broad-based it includes more than hands-on bodywork. Diet and nutrition, polarity exercises, counselling and reference to the types of constitutional types in the Ayurvedic model are used. The actual bodywork includes a wide range of techniques to rebalance and release blocks of energy in the body. This involves all the major systems of the body. The soft tissue may be manipulated, and pressure/reflex points used from osteopathy and chiropractic. This leads to a re-education of the body.

Benefits
Polarity therapy is particularly good for:

- digestive problems
- allergies
- ME and debilitating conditions
- stress-related illness
- back pain.

Contraindications
Cleansing diets, sometimes recommended in polarity therapy, are not a good idea for people who are very weak or ill, or for the very young or old. Active cancer needs to be treated cautiously.

Asha Christine is aged fifty-one, with one grown-up daughter. She was a single parent throughout her daughter's upbringing. She was so impressed with polarity therapy that she went on to train in it. She writes:

'I found the holistic approach (of polarity therapy) very liberating. At this time (1992) I chose to manage the meno-pause without HRT, which I had been taking in tablet form for five years. I received bodywork in gentle and deep pressure as appropriate. This released blocks that I had been holding.

Often I found that my posture and how I moved was different. I had to get used to my body being different. My mental patterns have also changed. I am less likely to panic. I notice when I am feeling stressed and help myself to slow down and be more positive.

Polarity therapy also gave me gentle exercises based on yoga together with using sound. These I do daily to continue releasing tension, emotions and holding patterns, thus providing more energy.

Polarity therapy has guided and supported me through cleansing and purifying diets so that now I understand why I eat certain foods and focus on what foods are beneficial to me at any given time. It has been quite exciting experimenting and really enjoying food. Over the past five years my tastes and diet have changed. I no longer eat meat, rarely eat fish or poultry and I am careful about dairy products because of the hormones that are given to cattle. A good proportion of my diet is raw fresh fruit and vegetables. In the winter I drink a lot of hot filtered water and all year try to avoid very cold foods. Since I did stress management training in the late 1980s I have not drunk coffee and I rarely drink ordinary tea these days.

Another helpful aspect to polarity therapy is the awareness that I have about myself and my environment. This means I am more in control and know that I can choose what I am and do with much more understanding.'

Kinesiology

In the medical sciences kinesiology means the study of the movement of muscles. Maggie La Tourelle and Anthea Courtenay write: 'Kinesiology is a system of natural health care which combines manual muscle testing with the principles of

TRADITIONAL CHINESE MEDICINE, energy balancing and other healing modalities. It is truly holistic, working with the inter-relationship between body structure, chemistry, the mind and emotions, and energy systems.'[12]

Applied kinesiology was created by George Goodheart, an American chiropractor, in the 1960s. The consistent diagnosis and treatment system he developed led to the foundation of the International College of Applied Kinesiology in 1973. For some time, he had been testing the strength of muscles to see if there was any difference before and after making spinal adjustments. This was done by seeing how well a muscle that related to the segment of the spine he was working on could resist his manual pressure. He found that particular sore points in weak muscles, once massaged, then tested strong. These reflexes or points that he discovered have later been called neurolymphatic points. Since the inception of applied kinesiology many new applications of the basic principles have evolved. These are collectively called kinesiology.

Applied kinesiology is used to detect incorrect joint function, muscle weakness, dysfunction of internal organs, spinal lesions, psychological effects on the function of the body as a whole, nutritional needs and allergies.

By studying healthy muscles that tested weak in certain conditions, Goodheart found that a weak muscle was often paired with a muscle that was in spasm. Usually we massage into the spastic muscle as a way of alleviating it, but Goodheart noticed that if he stimulated certain points to strengthen the opposing muscle, the muscle in spasm came back to normal alignment. Lori Forsyth refers to an analogy originally coined by John Thie: '. . . if a swing door is operated by two springs and one goes slack, the other spring will automatically tighten. Massaging the tight spring will do nothing to bring the door back into alignment — it is the weak spring which needs attention.'[13]

Goodheart found that muscles tested weak when there was structural misalignment but also when there were nutritional and emotional disturbances. He also researched the muscle meridian connection with Dr Felix Mann, a leading acupuncturist, and found that each muscle is related to an ACUPUNCTURE meridian. It then followed that through testing muscles he could find out whether the energy in a meridian was blocked or free flowing. Since each meridian relates to an internal organ, he could further investigate how specific muscle weaknesses can be an indication of organ dysfunction.

What is a muscle test?

There are around six hundred and fifty voluntary muscles in the body and about forty or fifty of these are frequently tested in kinesiology. A simple muscle test involves the practitioner applying a downward pressure of about two pounds in weight on the patient's extended right arm. On the instruction to 'hold', the person has to try and match the practitioner's pressure. If the person's arm locks in that position it indicates information is reaching that muscle unimpeded. If the arm does not lock and feels 'spongy' then there is some breakdown in the communication to the muscle. Specific muscles related to acupuncture meridians can be tested, giving an accurate picture of weakened muscles and their related systems. This is not muscular strength that is being tested, rather the neurological response, ie how well information is being communicated between the brain and the muscle.

A simple muscle test can be used to test the person's response – physical, emotional, nutritional, energetic etc – to any stimulus. The muscle must be strong to start with and tested to check that it is working properly and not frozen. Frozen means overfacilitated, which means it isn't functioning normally and is incapable of giving a switched-off response.

The muscle is tested while the stimulus is present. If the muscle remains strong this indicates the stimulus is not creating a stress. If, however, the muscle weakens this shows the stimulus is causing a stress. Having identified this, corrective measures can be taken.

How is a correction made?

Applied kinesiology and other kinesiologies use a range of corrections, some standard, others borrowed from other therapies. The person's body determines which correction will be effective. Standard corrections include the following:

- massaging specific reflex points to stimulate the lymphatic system
- touching reflex points on the head to stimulate the flow of blood to different parts of the body
- tracing the pathways of the meridians
- holding acupuncture points to stimulate the flow of energy
- offering energy-enhancing nutritional support.

After the right correction has been applied the previously weak muscle is retested and found to be strong, indicating clear communication between the brain and the muscle and also the meridian and its related organ.

When receiving kinesiology you are likely to be fully clothed. The number of treatments and treatment times vary, depending on the complexity of the problem.

Benefits

Kinesiology treats many illnesses that can not be helped by conventional medicine. It is particularly good for ascertaining food allergies or sensitivities.

Sarah is a middle-aged British woman:

'In 1995 I had what was at first diagnosed as an epileptic fit and was admitted to hospital for a few days, though it turned out that it wasn't that but an imbalance in my inner ear that affected my sight and consciousness. Following the 'fit' I was completely wiped out for a couple of months. I couldn't stay awake, eat certain foods without feeling sick, stand for long without feeling giddy or pick up anything heavier than a cup! My blood count had apparently been very low when I was admitted to hospital and, although there was nothing detectable in my blood, I was sure that I had some kind of infection as well as whatever had caused the 'fit'.

My acupuncturist was on holiday and some friends suggested I consult a kinesiologist, whom they described as a healer. I was sceptical, but so desperate for someone to tell what was wrong with me that I went to consult him. What an experience! He was like a clockmaker: elderly, courteous, perfectly practical. The consultation had some unusual (to me) features but, without touching me a great deal or any other examination, he was able to tell me things about my medical history that I had not told him on his first, very thorough, discussion and note taking. He told me that I had a viral infection that had embedded itself in my system. As well as the treatment that day, he gave me some exercises to do, which simply involved raising my arms in a particular sequence twice a day. Directly I left this consultation, I felt better; my face had colour and my partner commented on how well I looked.

As the kinesiologist had warned me, I felt a little unwell the following day but that was the start of my restoration to better health. His method is to ask the body when it needs another consultation and I think at that time it was in about three months. After that I went to see him about every six months, but now my body doesn't want to consult him for about nine months.'

Touch for health

Touch for health (TFH) was designed for the lay person to learn and use at home. It was put together by John Thie, who was a close colleague of George Goodheart. John Thie wanted to make techniques of applied kinesiology available to the public. So TFH can be learned in a series of weekend workshops. Participants learn how to muscle test, which muscles are related to which meridian and how the meridian system works, and how to give a treatment to balance the body.

Food allergies and sensitivities are usually tested by placing the particular food in the mouth and then testing the muscles relating to the stomach or other meridians. Such testing can determine which foods are life enhancing and which should be avoided or cut down.

The most fascinating thing I remember learning on a TFH course, which I did in the 1980s, is the ESR, which means 'emotional stress release'. This technique involves holding the forehead lightly in two specific places, halfway along the eyebrows and half way between the hair line and the eyebrows, with the fingertips. Beforehand the receiver has been asked to think about something that is troubling them and a muscle test will have confirmed this by a weak response. The receiver then continues to think about the thing that is troubling them and to stay focused on this while the forehead points are touched. The experience is that the problem tends to feel lighter after a time or even a creative solution comes to the person's mind. This can take a few or several minutes.

Lori Forsyth talks about her interest in how the mind and emotions affect the body: 'Using muscle checking and working from lists of possibilities, as well as using my intuition, I aim to pinpoint whichever of the life experiences of the client are a causative factor in the client's current state of poor health.'[14] She goes on to describe a new form of kinesiology developed by an Englishwoman called Chloe Wordsworth, called HOLOGRAPHIC REPATTERNING, which works on the vibrational resonance existing at the core of any trauma: 'When a trauma occurs, it gets lodged at a low level of resonance which is characterised by fear or anger or whatever survival response is triggered at the time and this resonance is returned to whenever a situation is experienced which restimulates the original trauma and the response to it. Whatever level the vibration, people attract and are attracted to those things and people which are vibrating at the same level, so frequently the low level is reinforced and a vicious circle is perpetuated.'[15] This sensitive work involves the use of COLOUR and SOUND as part of the treatment to restore the correct vibrational resonance.

Chapter Eight
The Metaphysical Therapies

The metaphysical therapies come from spiritual and esoteric traditions. As well as being firmly based in the concept of vital energy or life force, they are also founded on the belief that there are other sources of help for us in the universe. Throughout the ages people have felt and believed that we have subtle as well as physical bodies. This is reflected in the spiritual and philosophical writings and teachings of the ancient Egyptians, Chinese and Greeks, the indigenous population of America, many tribes of Africa, the Polynesian Kaunas, the Incas, the early Christians, the Vedic seers of India and the mediaeval alchemists and mystics of Europe.

It is therefore not surprising that today these therapies vary in their beliefs. Some overlap with religion, especially the traditional kind of spiritual healing in the UK, which can have a strong Christian influence with an assumption that a male God exists in heaven. However, there are many influences within metaphysical approaches, particularly from Eastern religions – Buddhism and Taoism – and from Jungian psychology. The concept of us each having a soul and there being a collective 'force' or 'consciousness' is more or less taken for granted. The term 'higher self' is often referred to by healers as an aspect of our being that we are aspiring towards becoming; a wise part that we can actually connect with consciously and be guided by.

Many metaphysical healers believe in reincarnation, other

dimensions and levels of consciousness where angels and spirit guides exist. This could be challenging if these areas of knowledge and beliefs are incompatible with your own. Psychic phenomena come into this category; telepathy, ESP and the changing of the molecular structure of the physical body through the use of the mind.

Practitioners of metaphysical therapies, and I include myself here, believe that we do not stop at our skin. We believe that as well as the physical body we have subtle bodies – emotional, mental and spiritual bodies – which to most of us are unseen. We also believe that 'reality' is multidimensional and that we can develop our senses to pick up information or impressions that are not normally available to us. This is often called the sixth sense, although who knows how far the human mind can really develop as our consciousness evolves. Everyone has the capacity to develop this sixth sense if they wish.[1]

Healing: subtle energy, auras and chakras

The following poem was created by Helen Williams after having been asked to explore 'What is healing?' in a 'Taking Root; Healing for Beginners' course at The Rowan School for Healing and Personal Growth:

What is healing?

A process . . .
A forward movement . . .
A realisation . . .
A transformation . . .

Wholeness . . . the search
for wholeness.
Freedom . . . to become

more of who we are.
A gateway where eternity
peeps through into time.
What is healing?

The next step that we
need to take along the
path towards our Selves.

Under this section I am using the term spiritual healing widely. Practitioners may call themselves spiritual healers, natural healers, psychic healers, subtle energy healers, bio-energy healers or therapeutic healers. Some healers prefer to drop the word 'spiritual' because it can be confused with religious or faith healing or spiritualism.[2] Spiritual healing can take place within Christian, spiritualist and other churches, but here it is part of worship and the expression of particular religious doctrine. It is an unpaid service, and the healing is usually received publicly within the congregation or 'healing circle.'

Some people experience dramatic positive physical changes through receiving healing. My experience was less so, but nonetheless important. For me experiencing healing was like 'coming home'. I discovered healing in 1980, a year after I had injured my spine. The healer I saw talked to me a little, very gently, then, with me seated on a chair, stood behind me and held his hands off my body, approximately two feet away. I was astounded. I could feel the same kind of sensations inside my body as I did on the osteopath's couch, but this man wasn't even touching me. I had a weird feeling that I knew about this phenomenon, it was familiar to me and yet completely new. I was hooked.

I had three sessions in all. There were no major miracles, but smaller, more significant ones. On one level I thought the healings were a bit of a non-event, simply because they were so uninvasive and because my healer was quite shy and said little. However, deep inside me I began to feel a new confidence, a new hope, and an awareness that there was a whole new world that I could step into. From a physical point of view it seemed as if these few healing sessions speeded up my recovery. I remember my osteopath being surprised at a later osteopathy session and he was able to do a treatment for which he had originally felt I wouldn't be ready for some time.

Anthea Courtenay writing in 1991 states, 'Healing is no longer a rather peculiar peripheral treatment, or a last resort for the desperately ill. The healing of minds and bodies and of the planet itself, by the laying on of hands, meditation and prayer, is being practised by thousands of individuals and groups.'[3]

What is it?
When we are truly still, quiet and relaxed – both in our minds and bodies – something rather special happens. We 'come home'. We stop, even for just a few seconds, and get some perspective on our lives and what is happening to us. When a healer lays on hands their aim is to help you relax. They also use themselves as a 'channel' for what they call 'healing energy'. They are seeing themselves as transmitters of life energy. A metaphor I use to try to describe this process is that of the power station producing electricity. This electricity is gradually stepped down in volume from local sub-stations through to the socket in your wall at home. If electricity came straight from the power station into your television set, the latter would blow. However, the television needs a certain amount of volts to do its job. So the healer uses herself as a small human generator. She doesn't give her own energy away (if she does then she gets depleted) but, through focusing her mind, she draws into herself universal energy that is then passed on to the receiver. As a by-product she can get a useful boost for herself.

Healing is also about connecting with the energy that is all around us. This same energy is constantly produced by ourselves as human beings. We are complex energy systems as well as thinking, feeling flesh and blood.

Auras

Healing is concerned with the balance of the subtle energy systems of a person. The healer may not necessarily touch the person's body, as she may work in what is called the 'aura' or 'human energy field'. This is an interplay of energies forming a field of energy surrounding each of us and has been shown to exist around all living things. For example, in the 1930s a Russian photographic technician, Semyon Kirlian, produced photographs by using high-frequency electrical currents instead of light and with this method was able to photograph this energy field. More recently I have had my aura photographed by a computerised camera. Through placing my hands on a sensor the electromagnetic field surrounding me could be measured. These measurements were then translated into colours based on the chakra system. Two photographs are taken at once: one of me sitting there and the other super-imposing the information from the sensor. Following this I received a polaroid photo of myself with the colours of my aura. These colours were then analysed by a trained interpreter. By having a photograph taken before or after receiving healing or meditating, or doing some exercise or whatever you can see the difference in your energy field.[4]

A healer is able to pick up the pulsations and vibrations given off by this energy field through her hands. By tuning into these vibrations a subtle shift of energy, usually a release or clearing, occurs in the receiver.

This idea of the aura or human energy field has been

around for a long time. Barbara Ann Brennan, an American healer and scientist, (she was a research scientist for NASA), uses the term human energy field as a modern scientific term for this phenomenon.[5] The aura can extend out from a few inches to several feet, depending on the health and vitality of the person. It is believed that in old religious paintings the halo represents the aura and many Byzantine paintings show this halo extending around the whole body as well as the head.

Many people see or feel this aura, often seeing or sensing colours. The energies within it are constantly in flux. Details of the physical, mental and emotional states of the person can be given through reading the aura with clairvoyance or clairsentience. With the former the healer focuses and concentrates on the quality of brightness, radiance or colour they can see surrounding the person. With the latter the healer scans the aura with her hands. Such sensations as heat or cold, density or depletion can be felt. Often there are tingling sensations in the healer's hands or the hands want to 'pull off' energy that feels congested or stuck. Various responses are felt by the recipient; usually they relax steadily and let go. The healer will usually scan the whole aura and then come back to parts that seem out of balance with the rest.

In esoteric psychology there are three planes to the aura: the physical, astral and spiritual. In books and esoteric teachings you often find confusion about definitions and there are variations as to how many 'subtle bodies' exist within these three planes. However, despite the different names and differentiations they all tend to work on similar principles, so that most healing will be helpful in a similar way. Here is one way of viewing them:

Physical: physical sensations, both pleasurable and painful
Astral:
• etheric: the blueprint of the physical body

- emotional: the emotional relationship to ourselves and others
- mental: the rational and intuitive mind working together

Spiritual: this involves a belief in a universal, benevolent intelligence, here referred to as 'divine'

- the divine will; connecting and co-creating with the overall evolutionary plan, ie that we are here for a purpose
- divine or spiritual love; includes spiritual/inspirational experience, such as being in awe or wonder
- divine universal mind; in a nutshell: 'be still and know that I am God', meaning having an awareness of being part of this greater intelligence.

Using this kind of model it becomes possible to diagnose imbalance long before an illness manifests itself on the physical level. Working with the aura can not only bring relief in the present, it is a form of preventive medicine.

Self-help
Here is an exercise to help you clear and balance your own aura:

Sit comfortably with your spine erect but not rigid. Use a cushion or pillow to support you if you need one. Close your eyes. Take a few deep breaths and relax. Take time to do this. Bring your focus into yourself and into the present moment. Now bring your focus to the space that is all around you – extending out from your body to about two or three feet. Sense this space above, below and to the back, front and each side of you. Now bring your attention to the space above your head and imagine that there is a beautiful golden ring there. This golden ring is like a huge halo and is big enough to contain your physical body. Imagine this ring very gradually moving down all around your body from the top of your head to the very bottom of your feet and below. As this ring comes down it gathers up any unwanted thoughts or feelings, or negative energy that you are carrying. It simply absorbs them. You may find your golden ring gets stuck in places and needs longer to 'collect' up the 'energetic debris'. Just let this happen. Don't force anything. Eventually it will come all the way down. Once this has happened imagine yourself wrapped up in a bubble of pure, clean white light. Stay seated as long as you wish and gradually open your eyes and bring your consciousness fully back into the room when you feel ready.

Chakras

Most healers, as well as practitioners of other therapies such as polarity therapy and yoga, also draw information from the chakra system (see Selected Reading). The word chakra is an ancient Sanskrit word, meaning wheel, and traditional Indian teachings depict chakras in a mandala-like design formed into a wheel or flower. Chakras are energy centres that can be seen clairvoyantly as moving wheels of light, and have different intensities, speeds and qualities, including colours and shapes.

This system helps us understand how vital energy enters, is distributed and leaves the human being, and this relates to each level of our functioning: physical, emotional, mental and spiritual.

These energy centres are not physical in the way that we may understand it, ie they cannot be seen or measured in the normal way. They are subtle, yet powerful, can be felt by sensitive hands and interpreted in a variety of ways. In exploring the chakras we use a map – rather like an astrological chart – that can help us understand where we may be under- or over-energised, where we may be stuck or vulnerable, where we may be centred and clear. Although each chakra and its associations are identified separately, it is important to remember that the system works as a whole and each centre is interdependent with the others. If one centre is malfunctioning then the whole system is affected.

There are many different interpretations, both in terms of location and the many associations made. These associations have included colour, sound, sense, element, evolutionary or level of human development, as well as the various components of the physical body, including the glandular system. Over the last few years other associations, such as gem stones, planets and aromatherapy oils, have been added.

The most common chakras worked with are the seven major ones, with secondary ones at the palms of the hands and soles of the feet. (It is said that each acupuncture point is a mini chakra.) On the physical level the chakras are located along the spine. The spinal cord, as a central organ of the nervous system, is the path along which impulses are sent from brain to body and vice versa. The chakras themselves are part of the human energy field, or aura, and are the main points of energy connection between the actual physical body and the non-physical.

Through meditation focused on the chakras, unconscious material can be accessed to be worked through and understood. It is as if the chakras are a gateway to our dream world. When we seek to understand emotional or psychic causes of difficulties within specific chakras we can help release physical problems as well. On a more day-to-day level, chakra meditation helps us to keep our energy clear and flowing. We can clear off energy we don't want, balance ourselves and consciously connect with both the earth and spiritual sources.

I have included a chart of these seven major energy centres with their various associations and appropriate affirmation. For further information refer to the sections on COLOUR, CRYSTAL and sound healing, AROMATHERAPY (Chapter 5), CREATIVE VISUALISATION and POSITIVE THINKING (Chapter 2).

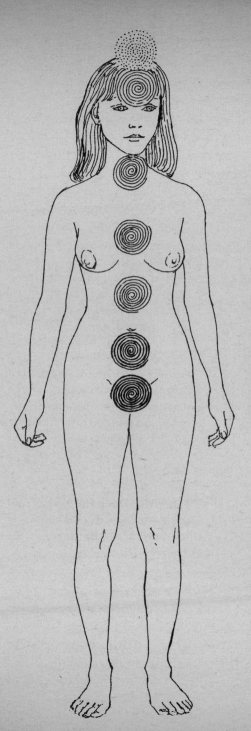

Crown

Third Eye – Brow

Throat

Heart

Solar Plexus

Sacral

Base or Root

Base or Root
In Sanskrit: muladhara

Gives vitality to the physical body

Location:	bottom of spine
Colour:	red
Element:	earth
Sound/mantra:	LAM
Musical note:	C
Sense:	smell
Energy type:	physical and raw energy, grounding and stability
Level of development:	survival of the physical self, primordial origins and conception, cellular level
Physical organs/body parts:	sex organs and organs of elimination (legs, feet and base of spine)
Gland:	adrenals (helps prepare for emergencies; 'fight or flight' response), gonads (sexual development; production of eggs in females and sperm in males)
Gem stone:	garnet, smoky quartz
Aroma:	cedar wood, myrrh, patchouli, vetivert
Planet:	Saturn, Earth
Affirmation:	I am fully aware of my position on earth and know that my basic needs will always be met.

Sacral
In Sanskrit: svadhisthana

Gives and receives energy for sexuality, procreation, physical vitality and absorption of food

Location:	back; sacrum and lower lumbar front; just below navel

Colour:	orange
Element:	water
Sound/mantra:	VAM
Musical note:	D
Sense:	taste
Energy type:	sexual, deeply ingrained habits, ritual, creativity, vitality, grounding
Level of development:	one to one relationships; the self and another
Physical organs/body parts:	also reproductive system, intestines, bladder, kidneys, lumbar spine
Gland:	as for base chakra
Gem stone:	citrine, amber, ruby
Aroma:	ylang ylang, jasmine, rose, sandalwood
Planet:	Moon
Affirmation:	I respect my needs and the needs of others in any relationship and will act accordingly.

Solar plexus
In Sanskrit: manipura

Vitalises the nervous system, and digestive processes

Location:	back; lower thoracic vertebrae front; diaphragm
Colour:	yellow
Element:	fire
Sound/mantra:	RAM
Musical note:	E
Sense:	sight
Energy type:	self-worth, self-esteem, social order and holding together own social group, prosperity

Level of development:	personal emotions and desire, being in a relationship with a group, being assertive and using one's will and personal power
Physical organs/body parts:	liver, stomach, gall bladder
Gland:	pancreas (controls level of sugar in blood), spleen (among other functions, stores blood and produces white blood cells and plasma cells[6]
Gem stone:	golden topaz, malachite
Aroma:	juniper, vetivert, neroli
Planet:	Mars, Sun
Affirmation:	I am worthy to live my life to the fullest, without fear or guilt, listening fully to my own inner voice.

Heart

In Sanskrit: anahata

Anchors the life force from the higher self

Location:	back; third and fourth thoracic vertebrae
	front; sternum
Colour:	green
Element:	air
Sound/mantra:	YAM
Musical note:	F
Sense:	touch
Energy type:	emotion; compassion for all forms of life
Level of development:	unattached love; accepting ourselves as we are
Physical organs/body parts:	heart, lungs, blood circulation; chest, breasts, ribcage
Gland:	thymus (growth, immunity)

Gem stone:	rose quartz, emerald
Aroma:	melissa, rose, bergamot, jasmine
Planet:	Venus
Affirmation:	I love myself and others unconditionally. I both give and receive love and respect my own and others' boundaries.

Throat

In Sanskrit: vishuddha

Gives and receives energy for speech, sound, and communication

Location:	back; lowest cervical and upper thoracic vertebrae front; hollow of throat
Colour:	sky blue
Element:	space, ether
Sound/mantra:	HAM
Musical note:	G
Sense:	hearing, sound
Energy type:	communicating, categorising, naming, channelling, self-expression
Level of development:	bridge between torso and head, spirit and matter; speaking our truth
Physical organs/body parts:	trachea, oesophagus, upper lungs, neck and voice
Gland:	thyroid and parathyroid (regulation of metabolism)[7]
Gem stone:	sodalite, turquoise, lapis lazuli
Aroma:	chamomile (German and English), lemon, fennel
Planet:	Mercury, Neptune
Affirmation:	I am willing to express my true self and therefore fully participate in my own creation.

Third eye – brow
In Sanskrit: ajna

Vitalises the lower brain (cerebellum) and central nervous system; affects vision

Location:	back; base of skull
	front; centre of brow, above
	bridge of nose
Colour:	indigo
Element:	mind
Sound/mantra:	A
Musical note:	A
Sense:	all senses plus intuition
Energy type:	rational and intuitive thought, imagination, perception, higher reasoning, idealism, decision making, clairvoyance
Level of development:	unlimited; only limited by the imagination or the intellect
Physical organs/body parts:	brain and medulla, base of skull
Gland:	pituitary (controls bone growth and regulates activity in other endocrine glands)
Gem stone:	lapis lazuli, azurite, fluorite
Aroma:	lavender, rosemary, juniper, thyme
Planet:	Jupiter
Affirmation:	I take full responsibility for my thoughts, words and actions.

Crown
In Sanskrit: sahasrara

Vitalises upper brain (cerebrum)

Location:	top of head, cranium
Colour:	violet
Element:	spirit

Sound/mantra:	OM
Musical note:	B
Sense:	extrasensory perception and beyond
Energy type:	spiritual awareness, wisdom, religion, higher aspirations, spiritual guidance, transcendence
Level of development:	oneness with all that is, beyond duality, truth, divinity
Physical organs/body parts:	cerebral cortex, top of head, cranium
Gland:	pineal (or seat of the soul, related to the regulation of the body's rhythms over an approximate twenty-four hour cycle)
Gem stone:	amethyst, clear quartz, diamond
Aroma:	lavender, frankincense, rosewood, jasmine, rose
Planet:	Uranus
Affirmation:	I am fully conscious of, and open to the will of, my higher mind.

In addition to these seven major chakras, there is also the upper heart centre (between the centre of the chest and the throat), the alter major centre at the bridge of the nose, and the identity point or higher consciousness, which is about eighteen inches above the head.

The aim of healing
The healer is concerned with the spiritual well-being of the receiver, not just with helping her physical difficulties. The focus may be on helping her to uncover the negative beliefs she has about herself on a deep spiritual level and to use this information to aid her healing process. Or it could be helping her come to terms with her situation so that she can live at

greater peace with herself. Many spiritual healers work with the dying, to help them end life in a meaningful way.

Unfortunately at the present time in the media or general public at large, healing is trivialised or sensationalised. The stereotype image of the healer performing miracles and the unrealistic expectations that this can bring is a major obstacle to receiving the genuine benefits of healing, which, apart from its deeply relaxing and de-stressing effect, is primarily about finding a place of inner peace and self-understanding. Physical miracles certainly can and do happen but they are rare and most healing is gradual and involves a commitment to change on the part of the receiver. Indeed, miracles come in many guises and many of them don't necessarily make good television or newspaper articles.

When you go for healing you will usually be asked initially to talk about what is bothering you. The healing itself will then take place either with you seated or lying down. You will be fully clothed, only removing your shoes and possibly any restrictive clothing, such as scarves or belts. Often healers use objects, such as candles or incense, to enhance the experience. They are likely to use soft, New Age music, although they should check if this is acceptable to you, as not everyone likes this kind of music. They will quietly attune themselves, which means they go into a very light trance-like state. They will still be very alert, but will have altered their brainwaves and will be in a meditative state. Their intention and compassion is important, especially as they are acting as a kind of transmitter or catalyst for life force. They will then work with their hands either on or off your body. Although the receiver does not have to believe that healing works, it does help if she is open to receiving.

The hands-on part of the session can last from anything from fifteen minutes to three quarters of an hour. Usually it takes less time to do a seated healing.

What can you expect?

Individual responses vary considerably, but the majority of people feel regenerated, relaxed, better balanced, more free of aches and pains and happier after a healing session. As with all holistic treatments, occasionally you may feel an increase in discomfort for a short time as adjustments take place or you connect with painful emotions that need to be experienced again before they are released. Often relief is immediate.

Healing does not conflict with any other form of treatment, either conventional Western, alternative or complementary medicine. You also don't have to be ill or in a distressed emotional state to benefit. It is an excellent pick-me-up and a way of maintaining balance and good health.

Benefits

Some of the effects of receiving healing can include:

- Balancing your energies so you feel clear-headed, grounded and energised afterwards.
- Experiencing pain relief, reduced muscular tension, a sense of well-being and relaxation. Your natural healing process can speed up.
- Feeling nurtured, supported and accepted just as you are.
- Connecting with a tiredness you have been ignoring and so may need to rest; also, as with all forms of hands-on work, you may become more acutely aware of areas of tension or pain and/or may feel some emotional upset as you connect with difficult feelings or unresolved memories. The healer needs to allow you the space to experience this.

Contraindications

There are very few. Care is needed not to over-energise people with serious heart conditions or those suffering with epilepsy. In effect, this usually means reducing the amount of contact time. Children may need to be worked with for a short time only (five to ten minutes).

It is important to note that, as with most therapies, you can experience an increase in the symptom(s) for a short time afterwards. This is part of the healing process and should not last for longer than a few hours at the most. Jenny, a woman in her fifties, describes her experience of this:

'I became conscious of a stiffness in my arm after the healing. I hadn't noticed it before. It felt like a shift of energy.'

Self-help

Because healing is natural and harmless there are numerous ways of helping yourself and many books available (see Selected Reading). 'Grounding is a word often used'. The idea of having our feet firmly on the ground and feeling that we are responding to external stimuli from the centre of ourselves is important if we are to feel good. 'Grounding' and 'centring' are useful awareness tools for both the healer and the receiver and, when I teach this topic in my own healing classes, people take the idea right into their lives and find it invaluable.

I often find it is easier to define grounding by describing what it is like not being grounded. When we are not grounded we will be scattered and/or obsessional in our thinking, disorganised, arrive at places too late or too early, be accident-prone and feel physically and/or emotionally off balance. The most extreme form of lack of groundedness is seen in the mental illness manic depression.

When we are well grounded we feel in touch with our physical bodies and feel that we are beings that are attached to the earth. We feel the ground under our feet, we feel stable, aware of the solid, core part of ourselves. We feel in balance. When we are grounded we are in touch with what we need. In my view all healing is about becoming aware of unmet needs (past and present) and finding ways to meet them. We all need help to do this and most of us are far better at seeing what others need than in seeing what we need ourselves. If we are not grounded we run the risk of projecting our own needs on to other people.

The symbolism of the Earth is important. The Earth nourishes and cleanses; it turns decaying matter into new growth. Our material resources come from the Earth and when we physically die our bodies return to her. Through connecting with Earth energy we not only use this for our own grounding, we can draw upon it and transfer its qualities to others.

The following are self-help healing techniques and are focused on feeling grounded in a healthy and balanced way:

- use your imagination: visualise a grounding cord, root(s) or rope going from the root chakra, or through legs and feet into the ground
- clear your own aura by imagining you are standing under a shower of beautiful white, cleansing light
- focus on your breathing; slow it down and be aware of its rhythm
- meditation: quietening/focusing the mind
- light a candle and focus on the flame
- body awareness – this means learning to notice subtle sensations in the body and respond to them, not ignore them. For example, a limb that needs stretching, a thirst that needs quenching
- eat a healthy meal with organic ingredients and drink mineral water
- rest
- use relaxation tapes
- do some tai chi; chi gung or yoga
- hug a tree!
- walk with bare feet on grass or soil

- do some practical tasks, such as gardening
- do some physical exercise, especially in nature; dance; stamp feet on the ground; lie on the ground under a tree; do drumming
- express and communicate thoughts and feelings and be heard
- be near water, especially the sea or a waterfall
- focus your eyes on a horizon
- get a bodywork treatment.

I recently received a healing because my back was a bit achy from having sat at my computer writing this book! This is what I wrote immediately afterwards:

'That was wonderful. I felt my back pain gradually lift off, like a helium balloon going up into the air, far away to the horizon.'

Dorothy, aged fifty-five, suffers from angina and received healing while on the hospital waiting list for open heart surgery. She describes her experience:

'I felt very uplifted and very relaxed as well. The pain in my chest was a lot better, as if the warmth from the healing had dissolved it like pouring warm water on sugar. When the angina bothers me I feel so depleted in energy. It's a horrible feeling. After the healing I felt as if someone had given me new batteries! I also felt very loved.'

Margo is in her early fifties, is black Caribbean, married and has two children. She describes how she combined spiritual healing with shiatsu:

'My psychological symptoms that led me to seek treatment were fear of the unknown and agitation. Also I was experiencing a moderate amount of back, neck and shoulder pain. I guess also I had feelings of self-doubt and lack of self-worth. I have been receiving spiritual healing for the past eighteen months, and I also have shiatsu treatment. I would certainly recommend these two treatments to others and have done. Spiritual healing has encouraged me to focus on myself and my surroundings. I am more aware of the 'now'. I am learning to appreciate myself for who I am. I am beginning to believe in myself more, therefore loving myself and everything and everyone around me.'

Therapeutic touch

'Therapeutic touch is a contemporary interpretation of several ancient healing practices. These practices consist of learned skills for consciously directing or sensitively modulating human energies' (Dolores Krieger, 1993).

'Dr Dolores Krieger is turning faith healing into a recognised science...' (*New York Magazine*). 'Therapeutic touch, first described by Krieger in 1975 as an act of healing or helping that is akin to the ancient practice of laying on of hands... goes beyond placebo[8] and involves an undefined but learnable method of human–energy balancing. In a world of expensive tools and high technology, human touch has been rediscovered as a valuable therapeutic method with dramatic implications'.[9]

Dr Dolores Krieger, professor of nursing at New York University, developed this form of healing in the early 1960s. She was invited to join a research programme that was being undertaken about laying on of hands at McGill University in Toronto, Canada. Dolores Krieger felt the laying on of hands could be useful for her student nurses. She realised, as I and many modern healers do, that anyone could be taught this skill, and that it had no religious connection.

This scientific interpretation of what is usually called spiritual healing has helped to make this therapy acceptable to the medical profession and the general public. I believe it is essential to demystify the whole business of healing, and Dolores Krieger's work has gone a long way to promote this. Through putting the framework for therapeutic touch into a nursing model, she began to teach it to her postgraduate nursing students in a programme called Frontiers in Nursing. By 1996 nurses in more than eighty universities in the US and fifty-three countries throughout the world were using this method. It was brought to Britain in 1989 by an American nurse called Jean Sayre–Adams and in 1995 was validated by the English National Board for Nursing. It is being taught at the University of Manchester to British nurses.

I did a weekend workshop based on the techniques and philosophy of therapeutic touch in 1982. Dolores Krieger had already published her book *The Therapeutic Touch* in 1979. I found it a simple, yet effective approach to working with subtle energy. The method provides a language in which to express rather abstract concepts, like auras and movements of energy. It has the same basis as ordinary spiritual healing in that the healer focuses her mind and makes a shift in consciousness. She is then able to repattern the receiver's energy into a balanced flow. The practitioner passes her hands over the receiver from head to toe, approximately two to four inches away from the body.

Techniques include preparing oneself to give by centring oneself and quietening the mind. The human energy field is then assessed. Different sensations can be picked up through the hands, differences in temperature being the most common. Other sensations of congestion, pressure or fullness can be perceived. There can be other clues, too: pins and needles, tingling, feelings of little electric shocks. The healer will also feel rhythmic pulsations in the energy field. These kinds of techniques are taught on many healing courses. However, therapeutic touch has developed into a form of its own with its own language and backup research.

As with other forms of laying on of hands healing, there is no need to undress to receive it. Sometimes gentle massage on neck and shoulders is done through the clothes to help relax the receiver, who is either seated or lying down. There is no standard length of time for the treatment. It can be as short as ten minutes, or thirty minutes or longer.

Jean Sayre-Adams states: 'Therapeutic touch can be viewed as an energy field interaction, the role of practitioners being to observe and repattern the energy field of their patients, therefore promoting relaxation and pain relief. The practitioner's level of consciousness would therefore be a central factor and, indeed, a part of the process is becoming "centred"; becoming mentally relaxed and focused on the patient'.[10] She goes on to describe the phases of therapeutic touch as being:

- Centring: the practitioner focuses on the here and now, disciplining her attention, achieving inner calm and establishing a state of receptivity in herself.
- Assessment: the practitioner uses her hands to determine the nature of the dynamic energy field. These are subtle sensations and are used together with perceiving intuitive and somatic clues.
- Clearing: here the hands are used in a downward sweeping way, just above the body, to facilitate the symmetrical and rhythmical flow of energy through the dynamic energy field. Research indicates that during this phase relaxation occurs and physical or emotional symptoms start to diminish.
- Intervention or balancing: here energy is projected, directed

and modulated. This helps to re-establish the order in the receiver's system and the energy field is repatterned. Energy is balanced and smoothed over areas of congestion and imbalance. The practitioner is part of this whole process and often relies on her own imagery or sense of imbalance to direct the flow of energy.

- Evaluation: judgment as to the completion of repatterning or rebalancing is made using informed and intuitive decision-making.

The modern physics view is that the universe is a dynamic web of interrelated events and that we and our environment are inseparable, and are the foundation of all forms of healing. Martha Rogers, also a nursing professor in New York, uses this theme in developing a theory of nursing. F Biley writes of Rogers' theory: 'This theory provided a radical vision of nursing reality which advocates a move away from a predominant medical model into a nursing model. The framework provides an alternative to the traditional view of nursing which could be described as Cartesian, that is, reductionistic, mechanistic and analytic, consisting of breaking up thoughts and problems into pieces and arranging these in their logical order. It has guided nursing out of a concrete, static, closed system world view and as a result has challenged many preconceived ideas about nursing and beyond'.[11]

Reiki

Reiki, Japanese spiritual healing, is an ancient and profoundly simple form of laying on of hands that is good for general well-being, relaxation and speeding up the body's ability to heal itself. It can be traced back to the healing traditions of Tibet and Egypt. As with the other systems it helps the mind to open to the causes of disease and pain, and helps the receiver take responsibility for her own life.

Reiki is derived from Tibetan Buddhism and, until recently, has been known only to a select few. It was rediscovered in the nineteenth century by a Japanese doctor, Mikao Usui. He sought the way Buddha healed. Some say he also sought the way Christ healed. He found the answer to his question in an ancient sutra (sacred text), which, unfortunately, has never been found. The story is that he was then inspired to meditate on a mountain, where he was shown a vision of four symbols that could be used for healing. As he came back down the mountain he stumbled and hurt his foot. When he put his hand on his foot the injury healed. As far as he was concerned his quest was complete. It is believed that these symbols activated the teaching in the sutra. Dr Mikao Usui passed on his knowledge and experience to others and two of them, Dr Chujiro Hayashi and Mrs Takata, were responsible for the way reiki has been brought to the West.

The actual word 'reiki' is made up of two words, 'ki' meaning life force, and 'rei', which means spiritually guided. It is a generic Japanese term for all life-force energy work, so is essentially the free passage of universal life-force energy. It can be used in conjunction with any other therapy.

The physical process of doing reiki involves a number of 'holds'; placing the hands gently but firmly in specific positions on the body. The body's energy channels are opened and cleared of obstructions by attunements. During this process symbols are used that reconnect you to your 'soul memory' and open you to access your 'Higher Self'. The receiver lies down and remains fully clothed. You can receive one or a number of sessions depending on your need. As with other forms of spiritual healing it is usually very relaxing and balances your energy.

Reiki practitioners go through an initiation process during their training. They are attuned by a reiki master and receive the healing power of the symbols. The term reiki master denotes teacher, reflecting the Eastern, apprentice-type, disciplined approach to learning, and involves the goal of self-mastery. The training is taken in three stages or degrees, and can be done in quite a short time. Some teachers teach reiki first and second degrees in just one weekend. Although this system of training may sound hierarchical, this is not necessarily so. You begin and then build on what you have learned. The training is essentially for self-empowerment and self-mastery. The symbols transmit powerful vibrational energies and the trainee needs to process the changes this brings to her life.

Again, as with other forms of spiritual healing, practitioners say that it is not they who are doing the healing as such. Rather it is the recipient who decides, perhaps unconsciously, how much healing energy they need or are willing to accept. What can happen is that you may aim to heal a physical symptom and find that it may not change, but that you no longer feel depressed or phobic about something.

Reiki practitioners do not claim miracles, although many people report great improvement in, for example, wounds healing, long-term depression lifting and tumours shrinking. Jane Alexander writes: 'At Stanford University in the US, reiki has been involved with a five-year project with cancer. Around three hundred people with terminal cancer, who had been given less than three months to live, were given reiki alongside their traditional treatment. After two and a half years, over half of them are still alive. This amazed the doctors, but what impressed them even more was the extent to which their quality of life had improved.'[12]

But nothing is predictable here. When the healing doesn't seem to work it is believed there is always a purpose behind this. Perhaps the person needs to stop for a while and rest.

I have some concerns about reiki healing, although it is clear that a lot of people get an enormous amount from learning, giving and receiving reiki. Although for the practitioner it is foremost a commitment to self-growth and a process that takes time, reiki has become very popular and some professionals have learned and are using the techniques very quickly. It could be seen as a seductive idea to initiate people, thus making them feel special and telling them they now have access to healing power. For those training in reiki it is important to learn with a teacher who offers the follow-up you need, such as support groups and supervision, when taking the courses. For the client it is important to seek a practitioner who has spent time processing and integrating reiki into her life.

I also have problems with the language. It seems so gender based; you proceed to become a reiki master. Although this reflects the oriental approach of apprenticeship, the term contradicts my belief that we are in a time when we are revalidating the feminine. I think one of the attractions and positive aspects of reiki is that it is healing with a name that has the attraction of being from the East, whereas the word 'healing' can be viewed as rather abstract and insubstantial, and words such as 'spiritual healing', 'subtle energy healing' or 'therapeutic healing' either imply religion (which may or may not be acceptable) or remain rather vague. I also wonder if healing in European culture is still associated with paganism, the occult or witchcraft in people's minds, unless it is seen as part of Judeo-Christianity. Fears and prejudices may not be far from the surface in people's minds. However, the popularity of reiki *is* resulting in healing, reaching far more people than perhaps otherwise would be the case. There is more than enough room for all these healing styles and traditions.

Here are some positive experiences of reiki:

After receiving reiki, Jane Alexander writes, 'Frankly, I was impressed by reiki ... In some strange way you feel touched by something very awesome yet infinitely loving. Perhaps it really is a divine blessing.'[13]

And Marilyn Kirby aged fifty-three writes:

'I found reiki treatments extremely relaxing and they sent me into a deep meditative state. The sky looked brighter when I left the therapist's house and I had a feeling of well-being. I now practice reiki on myself every day and for friends when they feel the need. I have also used it for emergency situations when people have been distressed. It has always, at the very least, calmed them and given them a relaxed feeling.'

Absent or distant healing

I describe this as prayer without the religion. Either individually or in a group, healers will focus sending love and healing energy to people who have asked for help. Group energy is stronger. Ideally you should know when the healing is to be sent so that you can stop what you are doing and focus yourself on receiving it. However, this is not always possible. Healing thoughts are also sent to the planet, the ozone layer, world leaders, people who are starving, children or adults in abusive situations, species whose existence is endangered and so on.

The simplicity of distant healing and naturalness of holding people you care about in your thoughts means that everyone can do this. There are a variety of ways of sending distant healing that can be learned. The most usual way is to relax and enter a meditative state and ask for help from whatever higher power you believe in. You ask that the person receive whatever it is they need for their highest good and for the highest good of all those connected with them. You then visualise the person well and happy, and that you are sending them love and light from your heart. The important thing is not to focus on what is wrong with them, or to try too hard. As with all healing at the end you close yourself down mentally, seeing your chakra centres closing or wrapping yourself up in white light. Some healers are trained to project specific colours.[14]

Laura Morton, now nineteen years old, was taking her GCSE exams when she was sixteen. She had been really struggling with the first exams and asked for some distant healing to help her. The healing was given at the time of her exam. Here's her story:

'I didn't realise until afterwards just how much more alert and confident when I was receiving the distant healing. I was able to sit down in the exam room and just do it. Everything just flowed and I wasn't so stressed. Before I'd sit and write nothing. I felt very lonely; in a mess. I'd tell myself "I can't do it." But with the healing I was very calm within myself and afterwards I was relaxed and not worrying lots about how I'd done, like I usually do. The healing was really comforting. I could feel it if I concentrated. I felt sensations of warmth, like someone was there with me giving me support, kind of giving me a little push to say you're okay.'

Radionics; holistic distant healing

This is a form of healing that can be done at a distance with the help of instrumentation: a 'black box' or biodynamometer. Treatment is given by directing energy patterns to correct imbalances. It is a complex therapy requiring training of approximately three years part–time study.

To understand radionics we have to look beyond biology and chemistry to quantum physics; a world in which matter and energy are interchangeable. In this reality all life forms are seen to be submerged in and interpenetrated by a common field of energy. The lowest levels of vibration of this field can be measured electromagnetically. However, there are many levels of energy that cannot be measured by scientific instruments.

It was Dr Abrams, an American physician, who developed the basic principles. At the end of the 1800s and beginning of the 1900s he became one of America's leading specialists in diseases of the nervous system. He identified the unique energy patterns of different diseases; this idea was far beyond the thinking of his time. Considering this to be an electro-magnetic phenomenon, he devised a box containing resistors, with which he found he could measure the disease reactions in ohms and so be able to distinguish one disease from another. For example, he found that cancer reacted at fifty, syphilis at twenty and tuberculosis at fifteen ohms.[15] In 1924 his basic diagnostic techniques were investigated by the Royal Society of Medicine and found to be 'established to a very high degree of probability'. It was an American chiropractor, Dr Ruth Drown, who found that it was possible to treat at a distance using a 'link' or a 'witness' between patient and practitioner. The use of a link, such as a hair or blood sample, is based on the principles of holography; that is, a small portion taken from the whole reflects the total energy pattern. This is like cellular biology, where each cell carries a copy of the master DNA blueprint of the body.

In radionics, as well as other forms of metaphysical healing, it is believed that any distortion in a person's field of life energy will eventually result in some kind of physical ill health. Radionic theory states that physical organs, diseases and remedies have their own particular frequency or vibration. As these can be given numerical values, called 'rates', and measured by the radionic instruments, underlying causes of ill health can be discovered and illnesses treated in their early stages.

As a form of vibrational medicine radionics is not restricted to time and place, which is why it can be done at a distance. Along with the ability to use radionic instruments, the practitioner will have a sensitivity to subtle radiations and so employs a form of extrasensory perception, often referred to as the 'radiesthetic faculty'. This can be done because the human mind, through the energy field in which it is immersed, can connect with the client no matter where she is. Along with asking a series of questions, this faculty enables the practitioner to obtain information about the health of the patient that is not directly accessible to the conscious, thinking mind.

Emotions and thoughts also have unique frequencies of vibration, as yet difficult to detect by modern scientific methods, but measurable with radionics. This therapy facilitates a flow of energies between the body's various levels to restore balance and good health.

Benefits

Many years of experience have shown that radionic treatment has been effective in alleviating if not completely eliminating the physical or psychological effects of both chronic and acute diseases.

Benefits can include:

- long-standing cases of asthma
- hay fever and other allergic diseases
- muscular and skeletal problems
- mental illness and stress-related psychological states
- digestive hypersensitivity.

Benefits often take a while to take place. Animals also respond well to radionic treatment.

Margaret Flavell is now a grandmother, and was a teacher. She leads a busy, active life. Here is her story:

'In 1987 I had a serious horse-riding accident that left me with only the use of my right arm. There was a lot of shock to my spinal cord but fortunately it didn't get severed. However, there was serious damage to my spinal column, pelvis and hip. I was hospitalised immediately. When I arrived at hospital they wanted to give me huge doses of Valium, which I refused because I wanted to be fully conscious of what was going on. I was told I would be in a wheelchair for the rest of my life and that I would need to take steroids permanently for the pain. I would not accept this. The doctors wanted to operate to fuse bones together in my back, and take bones out. I refused all the treatment except painkillers when I needed them (not when they were routinely handed out), and hydrotherapy (which involved being immersed in water). The latter started helping me and, although I was in a lot of pain, I began to feel in myself I could walk again.

Ten months later, when I was still in considerable pain, a friend told me about a radionics practitioner who lived five or six hundred miles away. I said, "How can this possibly work when I can't see this person and she's all that way away?" Anyway, I talked to her on the phone. She made no promises but said that conditions like mine had been helped with radionics. She sent me a medical and personal case history form, which I completed and returned to her along with a snippet of my hair. Our agreement was to stay in touch, which I did by both letter and phone. I needed to be willing to participate and be ready to receive the healing and know that something might come of it. At the same time it was important that I didn't give myself false hope or put pressure on the radionics practitioner to produce a positive result. My actual experience was that the pain decreased and it felt as if things began to go back into their proper place in my spine. I still use radionics to help my back.

Despite having been told I would be in a wheelchair for the

rest of my life, I've just been round the world with my new husband, climbed mountains, gone ocean-going sailing and horse-riding.'

Colour healing

Colour is a vital aspect of our lives and the colours we choose to wear or decorate our homes with influence us in subtle and often unconscious ways. The spectrum of electromagnetic energies that come from the sun includes the range that we experience as white light itself. White light contains all the colour frequencies of the rainbow. Electromagnetic energy is made up of sound waves, radar, microwaves, infrared light, visible light (the seven colours of the spectrum), X-rays, gamma rays and cosmic rays. These energies can behave as waves or particles. If we view this energy as travelling in waves then the longer the wavelength (the distance between successive waves) the lower the frequency (the number of times a wave oscillates in one second). The wavelengths of this energy vary and are reflected back to our eyes from the objects they strike. Our brains then interpret them as the various colours of the spectrum.

Colour provides a wonderful spectrum of vibrations for healing application; extremely fine vibrations ranging from oscillations of 436 billion times per second for red, to 731 billion times per second for violet. Violet is the highest vibratory rate visible to the naked eye.

As a form of energy, colour is active at all levels of our being and we all see colour in different intensities. Those whose vision is impaired are equally receptive to these energies, sometimes more so because they are more sensitised to non-visual stimuli. We not only absorb light through our eyes, we also take it in through our skin. Flesh is particularly sensitive to ultraviolet light. Theo Gimbel, the president of the International Association of Colour Therapy, says: 'Exposure to blue light over the whole body has long been a cure for children with jaundice, and ultraviolet light causes the skin to produce melanin (which gives us a tan) and Vitamin D (which is crucial for the body's metabolism of calcium).'[16]

The Ancient Egyptians are said to have built colour-healing temples. Sunlight shone through coloured gem stones on to those receiving healing. Colour is used in diagnosis in Chinese acupuncture, and in Europe colour was vital to the doctrine of the four humours: red blood, black bile, yellow bile and white phlegm.

In acupuncture the five elements – fire, earth, water, wood and metal – have associated colours. When the acupuncturist is diagnosing she will find out what colours her patient is drawn to or has an aversion to. Equally useful to the acupuncturist are the subtle colours seen in different areas of the face. This isn't just about skin tone; there are subtle hues of blue, yellow and green.

Each colour has specific effects. Our language again reveals this; we say we are 'green with envy', we 'sing the blues', we 'see red' when we are angry. On a physical level generally the red end of the spectrum makes the body tense, while the blue end tends to relax it. This is because red is a fast frequency of light and blue is much slower. Exposure to these two colours also increases or decreases the blood pressure respectively. Colour also affects our perceptions; for example, a red room feels smaller than a blue one. Emotionally, red excites us while blue calms.

Theo Gimbel again: 'Extremes of emotions are often the outward display of imbalances or blockages in the flow of colour energies into and out of the body. Analysis of these imbalances can reveal ailments before they manifest in the physical body, and colour therapy treatments, such as controlled exposure to coloured light, can adjust and correct the energy flow.'[17]

As with all the metaphysical therapies, the aura is viewed as a living phenomenon through which information can be perceived and interpreted. The colour therapist may use a pendulum to dowse the colour energies that are in the vertebrae of the spine and use charts to help analyse the illness and choice of treatments.

When the treatment involves using strong coloured lights to shine on to the patient, colours are used in their complementary pairs (turquoise is the complementary of red, yellow is the complementary of violet). The idea, as in POLARITY THERAPY and the yin and yang of CHINESE MEDICINE is that two opposites complement one another and create a wholeness, and also within the one is the potential for the other.

How does the colour therapist treat?

Correcting imbalances of energies inside the body involves the use of a number of techniques. These include full-spectrum lamps, coloured crystals, silks, and shapes, wearing coloured clothes, drinking solarized water,[18] using coloured oils in the bath, eating foods of specific colour, and the application of coloured oils during massage. Although colour healing can be applied in these ways, it is very effective to project the colours mentally. This involves choosing appropriate colours and directing them with intense concentration to the part of the body concerned. The use of the full-spectrum lamps is probably the most powerful of the techniques and therefore it is essential that this is done with a qualified practitioner.

Colour therapy helps the body to heal itself because the colours rebalance and revitalise the body's energies. There are colour therapists who work specifically with colour and a specific colour will be the medium for the healing. There are then healers who use colour as an adjunct to their natural healing abilities, so they may visualise colour as they do their laying on of hands (sometimes called mental colour therapy).

I do feel that because of the subjective nature of colour it is important not to make very hard and fast rules about what colours help what symptoms or states of mind. I believe that to a large extent we can intuit what we need and allow colours to come to mind that will help and support us.

Benefits
Colours are a powerful tool in treating the whole range of disease, for example:

- headaches and tiredness
- chronic disorders
- stress-related skin disorders, such as eczema and psoriasis
- depression, including seasonal affective disorder (SAD).

Qualities associated with colours
The following are some general associations. These vary depending on the healing system used and the preferences of the teacher. Most variations seem to relate to what colours to use for what chakra, part of the body or symptom. To my knowledge these qualities are generally accepted across the board. When working on children, highly sensitive or seriously ill people, use pale colours and limit the amount of time spent transferring mental colour energy.

Red
Energy, physical strength, courage, anger, inflammation, sensuality (deep red) and passion. Red-orange can indicate sexual passion, clear red moving anger, and dark red stagnant anger. Red can be used for charging the energy field and warming cold areas. It is used for blood-deficient diseases, such as anaemia. Too much red can produce rage or fiery conditions. Therefore it is not to be used where there is an inflammatory condition.

Orange
Vitality, joy, mental and physical balance, fertility and ambition. Also used for charging the energy field. Other uses are for increasing sexual potency, increasing immunity, and enhancing assimilation of nutrients, circulation and mental wisdom. It is the colour for the reproductive organs and the spleen.

Yellow
Wisdom, creativity, the intellect, fear and stimulating low energy. Used for clearing a foggy head and for increasing courage. Helpful for broken bones and bone conditions, as it helps to break up deposits (use with blue where there is inflammation). It is the colour for the pancreas.

Green
Growth, compassion, ingenuity, creativity, healing, envy and jealousy, pessimism, nurturing and harmony. It is a tonic for restoring frazzled nerves. Used for general healing and rebalancing the energy field. Spring green is good for some major internal organs such as the liver, lungs, kidneys, pancreas and spleen, because it cleans and filters.

Rose pink
Like green, rose pink is good for the heart. As a colour it is red with white. It is the colour for love, affection, kindness and hope. It is a comforting colour and is used to help ease trauma. It aids digestion, since affection is a form of nourishment. We use the phrase 'in the pink' when things are going really well.

Blue
Idealism, cooling, soothing, spirituality, imagination, inspiration, teaching, sensitivity, melancholy and motivation. Used for cooling inflammation, calming the nervous system and protecting. It is good for insomnia as it is calmative and

peaceful. Also used for pain relief, especially within deep muscle tissue and bone cells. It is the colour of the thyroid gland.

Indigo
This is the deep blue of the night sky. Movement towards a deeper connection with spirit, mourning, intuition, dignity and inner knowledge. Used for opening the third eye (of insight), and for quietening a busy mind. It helps with nervousness, mental disorders and transforming negativity. It is associated with the eyes, ears, nose and the pituitary gland.

Purple/Violet
Spiritual power and strength, deep spiritual connection and mysticism. Cleanses the energy field, and helps to connect and reconnect with higher self or spirit. It is associated with the brain and the pineal gland.

Brown
Reliability, moderation, solidity, capability and being down to earth. It is used for calming, for helping with concentration and for feeling grounded.

Black
Transformation, doorways to other realities and letting go completely in order to move into the new. Velvet black can be used to bring the receiver into a state of grace, silence and peace.

White
Truth and purity. Highly spiritual. Used for charging the energy field, for protection, bringing comfort and security, for pain relief and general purpose healing.

Silver
Communication and high psychic development. Used for reflecting back unwanted negativity, psychic protection and

strong charging of the energy field.

Gold
Pure knowing, intuition, connection to the source of life, service to humankind and strong protection. Used for strengthening and charging the energy field.

A note concerning serious illnesses: colour therapy is safe but would be used as an adjunct to other therapies.

Self-help
Self-help techniques include visualisation with colour and colour breathing. Here are a few exercises you can try. They were created by Kate Williams:[19]

Today's colour: lie down or sit comfortably with your spine straight and relaxed. Breathe gently and naturally; allow your mind to drift below your busy thoughts. Let the thoughts go. Ask yourself, 'What colour would really support and help me today?' Allow a tone or hue to settle into a steady picture or sense. Then imagine this colour completely washing over the whole of your body, making sure you include the areas above your head and below your feet, back, front and sides. Then imagine the colour penetrating every cell in your body. Do this until you feel satisfied. Very gently open your eyes and bring your awareness back into the room.

Colour breathing: this is no more complicated than visualising a specific colour as you breathe in and out. You can do it any time, any place, anywhere. Choose a colour that feels right.

Desk refresher: as you sit at your desk, imagine you are being bathed in a shower of white and gold sunlight. As this happens be aware of stress and negativity being washed away from you. Really connect with the sparkling white and gold energy and sense your inner being taking in the sparkling qualities of the white and gold, leaving you feeling refreshed and energised.

Jewel breathing, for anxiety: breathe in a colour of your choice, perhaps sapphire blue for soothing, or emerald green for cleansing. Imagine that you can direct your breath to the part of your body where you feel the most stressed; for example your shoulders or your stomach. As you breathe out, visualise the anxiety and worry flowing out as a murky mist. As you continue to focus on breathing your jewel colour, the mist will begin to clear and you will find you feel more relaxed and have a sense of inner peace. Repeat as often as required.

Circle of light, for fear: in any situation that scares you, as well as taking practical steps for your safety, surround yourself in a bubble of brilliant white or gold light to help you feel contained and protected. See the sphere extending above your head and below your feet, so the light surrounds you three-dimensionally and forms an invisible protective barrier.

Sound healing

Everything that exists is vibration, and as human beings we are affected by this, whether we are conscious of it or not. We exist within an ocean of vibration that is always moving, expanding, contracting and changing. Sound is vibration and can delight us, agitate us or heal us. Sounds cause different patternings in matter. For example, experiments done by Hans Jenny, a Swiss scientist in the 1930s, demonstrated how, when sand was placed on a metal plate and the plate was then pulsed with sound frequencies, individual sounds made the sand particles vibrate into particular formations. The very structure of life – genes, cells, DNA, atoms and elementary particles – all make harmonic relationships.

Music is a special type of sound. It is also a universal human language. Olivea Dewhurst-Maddock states, 'Music can bypass the mind's logical and analytical filters, to make direct contact with profound feelings and passions deep in the memory and imagination. This, in turn, produces physical reactions'.[20] The ancient Egyptians used music as long ago as 1600 BC to cure illness.

Incantations were used for cures for infertility, rheumatic pain and insect bites. It is said that the music of the lyre restored Alexander the Great's sanity in 324 BC. In the Old Testament King Saul's depression was lifted by David's harp playing. In Hellenistic culture, flute playing was believed to help ease the pain of gout and sciatica.

Lawrence Buchan tells us, 'The only difference between the vibrations of sound and the vibrations of colour is the rate of vibration; audible sound resonates in a range of 20 to 30,000 cycles per second, while colours vibrate between 400 and 800 trillion cycles per second. But the proportional differences between the seven notes on a scale and the seven colours of the spectrum are the same. Each colour has its corresponding musical note'.[21] Examples are: red/C, orange/D, yellow/E, green/F, sky blue/G, indigo/A, and violet/B (see Chakras, pp. 153–161).

Special sound frequencies are needed to bring about a state of well-being, and these are based on the relationships of the intervals between two or more musical notes.

Modern science is now helping to reaffirm this ancient knowledge. Olivia Dewhurst-Maddock explains: 'As the sound waves enter the body, sympathetic vibrations occur in its living cells, which help to restore and reinforce healthy organisation. The high water content of the body's tissues helps to conduct sound, and the overall effect is likened to a deep massage at the atomic and molecular level'.[22]

As with all the metaphysical therapies the sound therapist is working with energy: chi, prana or life force. Physical organs have their own notes and frequencies and vibrational energy is transmitted through the electromagnetic or 'morphogenic' field (the aura or subtle bodies) into the physical body. A healthy organ will have its molecules working together in harmony. There can also be a crossover with acupuncture, as the acupuncture points and meridians of the body have their own notes and frequencies.

The model of the chakra system is often used as a structure of energy centres through which the sound can pass. Each chakra vibrates at a particular frequency. When there is disease or the chakra is not functioning properly, sounding specific pitches into the human energy field can be a powerful way of correcting the vibration. Barbara Ann Brennan says, 'When I hit the right pitch, the chakra tenses up and begins to spin rapidly and evenly. Its colour lightens up. After holding the sound for some time, the chakra is charged and strengthened enough to hold its new level of energy.'[23]

Sound therapists use musical notations from different cultures, including Indian modes, known as ragas. Overtone chanting, with its origins in Tibet and Mongolia, involves practising the production of resonant sounds. A note can be separated into its octaves, rather like colour through a prism. You can work with a sound therapist to find your 'own note', which is your personal, unique, fundamental sound.

Benefits

A great deal of research has taken place in this field. Fabien Maman[24] is famous for working with sound to help disintegrate cancerous tumours. Others have developed apparatus for detecting and correcting imbalances throughout the body. A man called Don Campbell was able to heal a large aneurysm behind his eye by using the power of his own voice.[25] Other benefits include help with:

- premenstrual syndrome
- irritable bowel syndrome
- high blood pressure
- depression
- migraine.

Different musical notes have therapeutic applications. You can sing chants and mantras on the relevant notes and listen to music based on these notes. They indicate different senses, body parts, and pathologies. For example:

- The note C is concerned with the sense of smell, the bones and limbs of the lower body and blood haemoglobin. Singing C can help with poor circulation and blood disorders, cold feet and swollen ankles, lumbago, constipation or diarrhoea, urinary difficulties and melancholia.
- D is concerned with the sense of taste and body fluids, kidneys, bladder, lymphatic system, reproductive system, and the skin. This note is for asthma, bronchitis, gout, gallstones, obesity and detoxifying the body.
- E is for sight and the nervous system. It is related to the solar plexus. It is concerned with cellular repair, liver and intestines, and the intellect. This note helps with indigestion, headaches and skin conditions.
- F is about touch and feeling. It is concerned with the heart and lungs, shoulders, arms and hands, and also the hormonal

glands. This notes helps with hay fever, sleeplessness, irritability, high blood pressure and back pains. It can help to soothe emotions.

- G is about hearing and the area of the throat and neck. It is concerned with blood and circulation, the spine, metabolism, ears and the immune system. Conditions such as laryngitis, tonsillitis and throat infections can be helped as well as skin disorders, fevers and muscular spasms, including period pains.
- A is for intuition, all the senses and especially pain control. It can have a sedative effect and so help with all nervous ailments, including breathing difficulties and shingles.
- B is about the balance of minerals in the body and its fluids. This note helps with glandular imbalance and immune deficiencies.

A more general use of sound is found within psychotherapy. We often encourage clients to express suppressed feelings through the use of their voice. For example, expressing angry feelings safely using a bat and a big cushion rarely brings full satisfaction and completion without letting out the sound of anger in the voice. This can be in the form of yells, screams, grunts or words. Giving voice to frozen feelings is the way to dissolving them and freeing yourself. We sometimes need the chance to say, and be witnessed to say, something we were unable to say in a past situation.

Self-help
Body armouring – areas of self-imposed rigidity and tension – is described under the section on Reichian therapy (see Chapter 9). Certain physical conditions are the result of blocking in different parts of the body. Movement and sound therapy can help to release these blocks. For more detail consult Olivea Dewhurst-Maddock's book. If you are very anxious about what feelings may surface for you then only do a little, and make a

commitment to having some therapy if you can.

Here are just a few self-help ideas for difficulties in:

- The pelvic region; sexuality, menstrual cycle, constipation and feeling insecure. You may try moving to and listening to music that has powerful earthy rhythms, and sing while you do your chores.
- The diaphragm, waist area; you may suffer from ulcers, or liver or gall-bladder problems; you may be critical of yourself and others; this area is concerned with your personal power and self-esteem (see solar plexus chakra, pp. 157–58). Listening to, or singing along to, Handel's choral music may help; also sing near heat (if you don't have an open fire a radiator will do!).
- The belly area; particularly if you have an eating disorder, and general holding on to your emotional responses. Listen to string quartets and music by Ravel. Sing near water (in the bath or shower, by the sea or a swimming pool or in the rain).
- The heart and chest area; you may have lung conditions, such as asthma or bronchitis or you may have difficulties receiving love. Try listening to light music such as Vaughan Williams, and sing while outdoors in the wind.
- Throat area; you may have problems with hearing and your own voice, or you may be holding back on your creativity. Try listening to Mozart, especially 'Eine Kleine Nacht Musik'. Spend more recreational time doing creative things like painting, writing, reading and so on.
- Jaw area; you may keep getting colds, respiratory infections and migraines; you may be holding in your aggression. Try listening to 'Adagio for Strings' by Samuel Barber and start singing with others.

Sound within nature is known to all of us as a means of lifting our spirits. The market for healing tapes is very large and many of these tapes include the sounds of birdsong, waterfalls, fountains and the ocean. Visualisations can be added to what you hear; seeing the waterfall in your mind's eye significantly adds to the effect of the sound. You can imagine it washing over you, leaving you clear and refreshed. Since two thirds of our bodies are made up of water, this element is particularly healing for us. The sound and vision of running water is particularly good if we feel over-stimulated, or have pent-up emotions.

Remember that silence and laughter are also crucial to our sense of well-being. Silence can be a great comfort and needs to be treasured. Laughter nourishes sanity and actually releases endorphins – the body's natural painkilling substances – from the brain. It is said that a good laugh massages all our internal organs. Laughter makes us light-hearted and sparkling (see laughter therapy, Appendix II).

Crystal healing

Using a crystal for fortune-telling is one of the oldest methods of divination, practised widely in the ancient civilisations of the Egyptians, the Aztecs and the Incas. However, the psychic properties of the crystal do not stop with divination; it is a powerful tool for healing.

Crystals are an ideal energy source where healing is concerned. Much of the matter making up the human body is crystalline in nature so we have a natural affinity to crystals. I have found that children are very drawn to crystals. I was once at a complementary therapies exhibition. It was outside and breezy so I used a few large crystals to keep my leaflets held in place. Many children were attracted to them. They weren't interested in the leaflets! In fact crystal healing is wonderful for children because it is non-invasive and they can use their own intuition to choose the crystal(s) they feel will help them. A healer I know gives children who are in boarding-school a crystal of their choice to keep with them. In this way the crystal acts like a token or a friend.

Crystals work on the subtle energies of the body. Often the crystals are used as an additional tool to laying on hands and/or using colour. They amplify the energy and increase the power of what the healer is already doing.

Here are a few ways in which crystals are used for healing:

- The aura. A crystal is held in the left hand and passed gently over the part of the aura that corresponds to a physical pain or discomfort. While this is done the healer visualises the energy inherent in the crystal easing the pain.
- Direct contact. Crystals of various types can be laid on parts of the body – the recipient needs to be lying down. For healers who know about acupressure, it has been found that using crystals on appropriate pressure points adds to their effectiveness. Obviously the crystals need to have smooth edges so as not to hurt the skin. You remain clothed during the treatment and crystals can be used through clothing. Again the use of VISUALISATION by both healer and recipient helps to concentrate the positive energies flowing from the crystals to the troubled areas of the body.
- Indirect contract. The healer holds her own healing crystal in the left hand and rests the right hand lightly on the part of the recipient's body that needs healing. This crystal is a large, clear quartz and is used by its owner only.

However, crystal healing is an in-depth science and the properties of crystals are complex and cover a very wide range of problems. What works for one person may not necessarily work for another. It is best to build up a good knowledge of crystals and their properties and be guided by your own personal experience. Consultation with a qualified crystal healer is essential if you wish to use crystals for serious conditions. Here are just a few of the more common ones. Please note that these are broad guidelines only.

Agate
To improve vitality and increase confidence; good when you need a sudden burst of energy, eg running a race or taking exams. It helps you feel grounded.

Amber
For throat infections, bronchial disorders and those who are prone to asthma or convulsions. Amber is not really a stone but the fossilised resin of trees. It helps to clear emotions.

Amethyst
For psychic protection and for developing spiritual healing skills; it can help relieve insomnia and bring peace in times of grief. It is helpful for healing addictions.

Aventurine
For migraine and soothing the eyes. If you leave a piece in water overnight you can use the water the next day to bathe the eyes; also good for skin irritations. It is a comforter, and is also good for asthma and allergies.

Citrine
For poor circulation and to help control emotions; it can help with relieving energy drain, as in ME, and is good for mental clarity.

Coral
For facilitating intuition, imagination and visualisation; it is for stimulating tissue regeneration and for anaemia.

Jade
For kidney and spleen complaints, and yellow jade for poor digestion.

Lapis lazuli
Said to have the power to prevent fits and epilepsy and improve eyesight; it is for courage, wisdom and insight.

Malachite
Helps rheumatism, the immune system and irregular periods.

Pearl
For catarrh, bronchitis and chest and lung infections; it is peaceful and soothing, good for stress and easing childbirth.

Quartz (smoky)
An excellent general healer; it helps the development of mystical and spiritual gifts, freeing the mind from unwanted thoughts. Rose quartz is good for migraine and general headaches.

Rose quartz
Encourages genuine self-love, helps free us from worry; it stimulates blood circulation, fortifies the heart and helps with fertility.

Sodalite
Blue sodalite is useful for assisting the lowering of blood pressure and for cooling fevers or high temperatures; for thyroid conditions.

Tiger's eye
Helps counteract the fear of becoming ill; good for reproductive disorders.

Topaz
Also for high blood pressure and reducing varicose veins; it revitalises, and helps with ear, nose and throat problems, the liver and gall bladder.

Tourmaline
For relief of nervousness and encouragement of self-assurance; helps release old emotional pains and fears. It is good for the heart, thymus and immune system. Black tourmaline is for protection from radiation.

Turquoise
Among Native American people it is believed that it absorbs harmful vibrations; at one time it was frequently given to people about to undergo surgery as a form of protection. It is a very spiritual stone, and helps heart, lung and throat conditions.

Crystals need to be cleansed regularly because they absorb a great deal of negative energy. For example you can wash them in cold water, preferably cold running water. However, don't do this for coral or lapis lazuli because they are porous and so will absorb the water rather than be cleansed by it. All the crystals mentioned here can be cleaned and cleared by being placed in direct sunlight or moonlight. Some crystals like to be buried in soil or kept in a dark cloth or pouch, but most crystals like light.

When choosing a crystal among several you might like to close your eyes and visualise your ideal one. When you open your eyes, pick up the first one you are drawn to. Or you can hold your hand over the crystals and if you feel a slight magnetic pull, or a tingling sensation over one particular crystal, this means that your energetic vibrations are compatible. This will be the one that can help you at that time.

Because crystals are easily available, this is a therapy that is accessible in the form of self-help. However, crystals need to be handled with care. If in doubt as to how to use them consult a qualified practitioner (see Resources).

Self-help

- I have a large piece of smoky quartz on the monitor of my computer. I think it helps protect me against the effect of electromagnetic radiation coming from the screen. It also is the crystal for helping you get work done, resist stress and concentrate. Physically it helps dissolve cramps, and is particularly good for back pain.
- If you have a headache hold a gentle coloured crystal against your temples or on or around the affected area. For example, you could use rose quartz or aventurine.

Chapter Nine

Body Psychotherapy, including Rebirthing and Hypnotherapy

Psychotherapy is a large and complex field of theories, treatments, research and experience. It has proliferated considerably since it began in its modern form with Freud's 'discovery' of the unconscious in the late nineteenth century. Although its forms are diverse, underlying many kinds of psychotherapy is a belief in the value of empathy, warmth and acceptance, and careful attention to how the client feels, her state of mind, the way she behaves, and how she forms and maintains relationships.

All of us have parts of ourselves and our lives that we feel satisfied with and other parts that we don't. The latter may be difficulties in communication with others, conflict in our families or the workplace, feeling confused, anxious or unfulfilled. The function of any kind of personal development work is to bring a spotlight to the areas of our lives that are not working for us, so that we can see them more clearly and develop new skills and choices in dealing with them. Some psychotherapeutic approaches are specifically body oriented and there is now a category, called body psychotherapy, which encompasses many different types of therapies (see also Appendix II for short descriptions of some of these therapies that have not been included in this chapter, ie core energetics, energetic integration, Hellerwork, holotrophic breathwork, psychomotor, radix, somatic emotional therapy). These approaches are often available in psychotherapy centres that define themselves as being humanistic and integrative.[1]

Any form of psychotherapy that helps us emotionally and mentally may help us physically. However, body psycho-therapists use bodywork to encourage the client to feel safe and contained, and to support the process of becoming open to powerful feelings and conflicts that we learn to repress and suppress over a lifetime. Through this work the client can feel more alive and spontaneous, and develop a greater trust in her own body and what it is telling her.

Stanley Keleman, director of the Center for Energetic Studies in Berkeley, California, writes '... the form and the movement of my bodily expression reveal the nature of my existence... I am my body. My body is me. I am not a body; I am *some*-body.'[2]

We shape our bodies throughout life through our feelings and our responses. My body isn't an object in space, it is the embodiment of me as a person. The ways in which we hold ourselves and move reflect our experiences and attitudes. These in turn have often been shaped by cultural influences; our families and society. As children we all needed to grow both physically and emotionally, to cope with and survive all the problems and challenges of our childhood. Some of our survival strategies continue to work well in adulthood; others may bind us in repetitive and sometimes destructive patterns of behaviour.

As body psychotherapists we constantly work with the notion of the body–mind as an energetic matrix reflecting the person's life history, and the recognition that psychological wounds are carried and remembered in the body... In particular, we recognise the activity of the autonomic nervous system as a barometer of an individual's conscious and unconscious reactions to experiences... The autonomic nervous system effects breathing, digestion, contraction and relaxation of muscles, blood circulation, the production of certain hormones – such as adrenalin – and the immune system. It produces changes in the body that reflect an individual's thoughts and feelings, but which often occur outside awareness.[3]

In general within psychotherapy it is the emotional and psychological contact between the client and the therapist that is considered to be the vehicle through which positive change for the client takes place. This is very different from the 'hands-on treatment' kinds of therapies described elsewhere in the book. Body psychotherapy particularly is not a technique or a treatment 'done' to the client. Any techniques used are an integral part of a therapeutic relationship. As Bernd Eiden says, 'Real change only happens through relationship with another human being, because the original damage and consequent formation of habitual patterns occurred in the dynamic with people in an individual's early environment'.[4]

As part of their work, psychotherapists often work with the dynamics of **transference** and **counter-transference**. Since these words have entered popular language, I think it would be useful to give a full definition here. This can help explain how some aspects of the psychotherapeutic relationship work. Transference refers to an emotional attitude, positive or negative, felt by the client towards the therapist. The client is experiencing something that she has felt before in a different situation – usually with parents, carers, school teachers or others in positions of authority over them – and they are now transferring this experience inappropriately to the present situation. As a client, you will bring with you to the therapy situation your history of behaviour. People often choose to go into therapy because they want to understand why they behave in ways that are repetitive and prevent them having the kind of life and relationships they want.

Transference and counter-transference are usually an integral part of the psychotherapeutic process. The role of the therapist is to receive this transference and help her client see that not everyone is going to respond to her or view her in the same way her parents or carers did. For example, if your mother was a very critical person (usually because her mother had been, and so on, back through the generations), it is likely that you will expect other women in positions of authority to be critical of you; in this situation your female therapist. This is called negative transference. When you start relating to your therapist as if she were your mother – perhaps you feel irrationally fearful or angry – your therapist can help you untangle the transference. The part of you that actually still feels like a child when with a woman in authority can choose to have a different experience, heal, and so become more comfortable with being in your own authority and your personal power. Working with an appropriate male therapist potentially supports a woman to heal her relationship with her father.

Counter-transference occurs when the psychotherapist develops an emotional attitude towards the client based on the psychotherapist's own past. This is something the psychotherapist must watch out for. For instance, if she too had a critical mother, she may fall in to the trap of starting to behave like her own mother, and by definition possibly like the client's mother, too. This is why if you are seeking psychotherapy it is essential that you work with someone who is professional, mature, has integrity and good supervision (see Chapter 4).

Positive transference is when you, as the client, view your psychotherapist as an ideal, superhuman kind of person who is all wise and all knowing. Here part of the therapeutic process for you would be to learn that she is indeed human. She has good days and bad days, just like you; she has nice parts of herself and nasty parts of herself, just like you; and is working on her own self-healing, just like you. In this situation the task of the psychotherapist is to see what is happening and not collude with your need to constantly tell her how wise she is. It is also part of her job to help you learn to see that you have a lot of wisdom about your own process and needs.

The concepts of transference and counter-transference connect with the term **projection**. We project when we attribute to a person, situation or object outside ourselves the feelings or thoughts that actually belong to us. This is usually an unconscious process. We all do this in order not to live the experience of these feelings or thoughts. Such feelings or thoughts may be negative or positive; eg guilt, anger, sadness, prejudice, or excitement, admiration or joy. One of the tasks of the psychotherapist is to watch out both for the client's projections on to them and vice versa. An example of projection would be thinking that somebody is angry with you, when in fact it is you who is angry with them.

The history of body psychotherapy

Wilhelm Reich is described as the father of most present-day body-oriented psychotherapies. Born in 1897, he was an Austrian psychoanalyst who was a clinical assistant to Sigmund Freud for six years in Vienna. But in 1933 he broke away from Freud; he was critical of psychoanalysis and its slowness to bring about change, disregard of body language and taboos on touch. His theories were controversial, and pioneering in relating neurosis to a physiological basis. In 1939 Reich settled in the US, when he began his work with orgone energy. This is yet another term for prana, chi or life force. Reich referred to orgone as cosmic energy that can be seen and measured and that exists in all living organisms.

Whereas psychoanalysis was, and is, largely verbal and

insight oriented, Reich developed a system of therapy that works directly with the body, using a wide range of techniques to release repressed sexual-emotional energy. Richard Hoff describes this: 'The ultimate aim of the therapy is to dissolve neurotic character structure and muscular armouring at the deepest biological levels, to restore free, natural energy flow, and, finally, to establish "full orgastic potency" – the ability to build and release full energy at the moment of orgasm.'[5]

Reich believed that, because sex was enshrouded in secrecy and associated with obscenity, shame and guilt, we learned to fear and resist our deepest natural urges and contract the whole of our being in order to suppress spontaneity and aliveness. He used the word armouring to describe how we chronically contract our bodies to suppress not only our natural life-energy flow but also the frustration and pain that results from this suppression. Vegetotherapy is the term he used to describe his method of softening muscle tensions and deepening breathing so as to release blocked emotions and recover a sense of pulsation and streaming in the body.

Reich developed 'character analysis', which involved focusing on the 'how' of a person's behaviour. For example, how a person speaks – her voice quality, intonation and expression – is as significant as what she is actually saying, if not more so. This focusing on the process – the 'how', rather than the content of 'what' we say or do – is essential to other psychotherapies too, especially GESTALT (see p.214). When we develop awareness we gain insight into the meanings of habitual behaviour; posture, gait, mannerisms, gestures and facial expressions. Our stories are contained in these characteristics. How we have psychologically adapted to life events can be seen in our bodies and how we move.

Reich found that repressed emotions are physiologically rooted in chronic muscle spasms. Emotions are not just feelings that float in our brains; every emotion involves an impulse to action. For instance, if we are sad, we have an impulse to cry. Crying is a very physical event and involves bodily changes such as a kind of convulsive breathing, tears, vocalising, facial expressions and often limb action. When we suppress the urge to cry we also have to suppress all those muscular impulses. Most especially we hold our breath.

Suppression turns into repression when the inhibition of expression of emotion has become so habitual it turns into chronic muscle contraction and this becomes automatic and unconscious. This kind of tension cannot be voluntarily relaxed, even in sleep. Reich says that these forgotten memories and feelings lie dormant, but intact, in the muscles in the form of 'frozen impulses to action'. The flow of vital energy throughout our bodies becomes blocked. These blocks he called 'armouring'. He identified seven major segments of body armouring, beginning with the eye segment and continuing down through the body via the mouth, neck, chest (including the arms), the diaphragm, abdomen to the pelvis (including the legs).

Reich developed many techniques to help to dissolve this muscular armouring. These include:

- deep breathing, and vocal and physical expression of emotion (including screaming)
- deep massage used on the tense areas, with the client breathing deeply and vocalising at the same time
- work with facial expressions
- pushing down on the chest while the client breathes out
- work with the 'gag reflex' (the yawning or cough reflex); any convulsions tend to help break down the rigid armouring and these can reach deep internal armouring that would otherwise be inaccessible
- maintaining 'stress positions' especially while breathing deeply and expressing the pain with voice and face

- active 'bioenergetic' movements, such as pounding, stamping, kicking, reaching out, and moving or shaking areas such as the head, shoulders, arms or pelvis.

Reich's therapeutic work and research was taken up both in Europe and the US by many of his followers. These therapists have then developed independent, distinct and varied approaches. These include BIOENERGETICS, BIODYNAMIC PSYCHOTHERAPY, HAKOMI, biosynthesis and core process. Over the last twenty-five years body psychotherapy has considerably refined its techniques and now employs more subtle ways of working with more attention to what is taking place within the relationship between therapist and client. Ways of working may include different modes of relating. The therapist may sit with the client face to face, or the client may lie down on a treatment couch or a mattress. At times the client may be encouraged to stand or move (see Chapter 10).

The therapy work needs to start with the most superficial defences and work gradually into the deeper layers, and the client's fear and resistance should always be respected. We build up this armouring as part of our emotional survival as we grow up and any 'undoing' or disorganising needs to be done with great care.

This whole process of dissolving body armouring, together with character analysis, requires courage, perseverance and support, both from the therapist and close, loving relationships. We not only need to learn to release emotion, we also need to allow love and support in. It is essential to always work with a properly trained therapist who has her own professional supervision for her work.

Neo-Reichian therapies are more recent developments of the work of Wilhelm Reich. What they share is a continued focus on the body as a means to contact the impulses towards aliveness and well-being, as well as survival strategies learned early that restrict our spontaneity and joy. What they also share is a new focus on the interpersonal arena (the family, school and community) in which bodily patterns get established and are maintained, and the more spiritual (often called trans-personal) context in which we are all seeking purpose and meaning in our lives. Moreover, most neo-Reichian therapies will differentiate between armouring caused as we develop and that caused by trauma, and the therapist will use different techniques of working with the different body processes involved.

Bioenergetics

This therapy was developed out of Reichian bodywork by an American doctor called Alexander Lowen, together with John Pierrakos. Lowen studied with Reich throughout the 1940s. Whereas Reich followed the psychoanalytic tradition in having his patients lie down during sessions, Lowen started to work with his patients standing. He stressed the need to bring the legs to life and establish a firm connection with the ground. He also emphasised sexuality less than Reich, viewing it as just one of several bodily drives including moving, breathing, feeling and self-expression.

Lowen describes bioenergetics as a therapeutic technique to help a person get back together with her body and to help her enjoy the life of the body to the fullest degree possible. In a therapy session the client will relate her history and what she would like help with. The therapist then studies her bodyform, its movements and the sound of her voice in order to find out where and how her emotion is held. The work may include the client being encouraged to stand in 'stress positions', such as standing as if sitting on a chair. This forces the muscles to surrender and to shake off tensions. A combination of breathing exercises, stretching or expressive exercises may be used to help release tension. Exercises that can be done by the client at home are taught, if this is appropriate. This kind of work is carefully done in cooperation with client and therapist.

Elaine Stillerman points out, 'In bioenergetics it is important to keep in mind that any limitation of movement is both a cause and effect of emotional problems, and any restrictions of natural respiration are both a cause and effect of anxiety... In bioenergetics, the physical tension is released concomitantly with the psychological.'[6]

Hakomi

The word 'Hakomi' is ancient Hopi (Native American). Its literal translation is 'How do you stand in relation to these many realms?' or, more simply, 'Who are you?' Hakomi is a body psychotherapy that supports the client to revise her core beliefs. These beliefs are the ones that are self-limiting and were formed early in life and stored in the subconscious mind. These beliefs, such as 'I am not good enough', 'I am unwanted', involved certain feelings, thoughts and sensations powerful enough for the child to create a set of ideas about herself. The therapy traces back through childhood events to the origins of the child's responses. It assists the client in focusing on and studying how she organises these core experiences; she may recapture an experience and feel it in her body. She is then able to change her reaction to the experience.

The Hakomi method was developed by Ron Kurtz in the late 1970s. He was influenced by FELDENKRAIS, GESTALT, BIOENERGETICS, ROLFING, REICH, ERICKSONIAN HYPNOSIS, neuro-linguistic programming, as well as the traditional Eastern philosophies of Buddhism and Taoism. This is an inclusive therapy and continues to be so. The Hakomi therapist recognises the value of and encourages the use of other help for the client, such as nutrition, cranial work (eg see CRANIAL OSTEOPATHY, CRANIO-SACRAL THERAPY) and structural or movement work (eg see POSTURAL INTEGRATION, DANCE MOVEMENT THERAPY). The Hakomi method, like so many others, reflects the new paradigm; the movement away from the reductionist, mechanical linear model towards a model of interconnectedness, of multiple possibilities and greater complexity (see Chapter 1). Hakomi therapist Emerald-Jane Turner states, 'There are many different ways to approach the places in ourselves that have been frozen in time, each one valid in its own right.'

Ron Kurtz defines five principles of the Hakomi method:

- organicity: this means that healing involves natural processes; as individuals we grow and unfold. All the answers and resolutions to our problems are within ourselves
- body-mind holism: the recognition that mind and body interact and influence each other
- non-violence: this means acceptance and attention to the way things naturally want to unfold. The therapist must let go of her own ideas — her agenda — about what she may want for her client
- unity: this is about bringing attention to aspects of ourselves and others that are in isolation or conflict; we are connected to each other and the world
- mindfulness: focusing on present experience.

A prime aspect of the work is that the client needs to feel emotionally safe, and that in order to focus on what she feels in the present there is a need to slow down. Hakomi therapy works at the body-mind interface. It is body centred in that it recognises the importance of working with and acknowledging the information from the body. Posture, gestures, body structure and subtle habitual movements are highly significant in that they are directly connected to thoughts, memories and belief systems. As a client these bodily aspects of yourself are studied by both your Hakomi therapist and, with her help, yourself.

Hakomi therapy is done during an altered state of consciousness called mindfulness, a place of acute awareness and deep knowing. Elaine Stillerman says, 'Mindfulness encourages open communication between the conscious and unconscious minds. It is possible for an individual to observe [her] experiences without interference or judgement. The therapy is an exploration of the limiting choices a person has made and provides [her] with the ability to make new, self-affirming ones.'[7] This process also helps the client to re-establish contact with her talents and strengths, not just her limiting beliefs or negative experiences.

The Hakomi therapist does not give advice, try to solve problems or encourage her client to talk about the past. By paying special attention to safety and slowing down the thinking and feeling process, material from the client's unconscious emerges. The therapist goes to the client's body-mind for information. For example, if a client has issues about her sister, the therapist will ask questions such as 'So where in your body does that difficult feeling resonate right now?' Or the therapist may ask her client to find the sensation that goes with a thought, memory or issue. This is done through talking. Touch is only used with the client's permission and within the context of mindfulness and the particular issues they are working on. The therapy tends to be long term. You may have weekly or fortnightly sessions for up to two years. It takes time to dive into the depths of one's being and then live and embody the Hakomi method principles.

Contraindications

Hakomi therapy is not suitable for people who are very agitated or seriously depressed. Although you don't have to know about mindfulness or be able to do it before you begin therapy, you do need to have the ability to access it. If your distress is extreme you are unlikely to be able to slow down or centre yourself sufficiently to experience mindfulness.

Celia West is forty-six years old and has cancer. She now lives in New Zealand. Celia is an example of both the interconnectedness that Hakomi has with other therapies and the life-giving power of handling 'the chasm', integrating both orthodox medicine and CAM. In order to help keep herself alive she uses a balance of chemotherapy from orthodox medicine and a number of different CAM therapies, such as subtle energy healing, Chinese herbs, acupressure, art therapy and nutritional therapy for cancer. This is her experience of Hakomi therapy:

'I grew up in New Zealand but lived in England for many years, where I completed ten years of psychotherapy (five years neo-Freudian, and five years of gestalt). I started seeing a Hakomi therapist after returning to New Zealand in 1993 because, after being away so long, I was unable to reorient myself in terms of who I was in relation to the culture and how I could fit in. Just after beginning Hakomi therapy in November 1995 I was diagnosed with acute leukaemia. After two initial rounds of chemotherapy the hospital considered there was nothing they could do for me.

It was shortly after my diagnosis that I had an extremely important experience during the Hakomi therapy. It's hard to describe but I was in an almost meditative state. The therapist uses what they call 'probes', which are messages to you when you're in this meditative state. Hakomi therapists call it mindfulness. I suddenly had an experience of letting go, relaxing, trusting and receiving from this therapist in a way I had never experienced before. It was about really healing a deep wound around trust. I stopped a lot of my internal struggle and had a lot more peace around the process I was going through with the cancer. In talking about healing in a non-curative sense I think the cancer was partly engendered by that struggle and, although I still have cancer, the hospital staff don't know how I've survived so long. Now, four years on, I am not a survivor of cancer; I am not a victim of cancer. I am living with cancer. I have made my peace with it. The hospital staff say, "We don't know what you're doing, but you must be doing something right. Keep doing it!"'

Biodynamic psychotherapy

Biodynamic psychotherapy emphasises and directly addresses the energetic and emotional meaning of physical posture and bodily symptoms. It is based on physical, emotional, mental and spiritual dimensions of existence.

It was developed by Gerda Boyeson, who was a clinical psychologist, physiotherapist and psychotherapist in Norway. She brought it to England in 1968. 'Bio' means life and 'dynamic' means movement or forces and so, central to the work is the idea of life movements and re–establishing a natural flow of them in the body. As with BIOENERGETICS and GESTALT THERAPY, Boyeson was also influenced indirectly by the work of Wilhelm Reich. She had analysis with Dr Ola Raknes, who was part of Reich's circle in Scandinavia in the 1930s. Gill Westland, director of the Cambridge Body Psychotherapy Centre, says '... alongside access to the unconscious through the use of words, it is possible to work directly with the body through massage, breathing, and movement. Changes in the body are accompanied by psychic changes...'[8] So Boyeson became convinced of the importance of working both verbally and bodily.

A main theory in biodynamic psychotherapy is that energy moves constantly through cycles: the 'vasomotoric cycle'. However, these energetic cycles often get interrupted and remain incomplete, so the therapist works to encourage completion. For instance, if I'm crossing the road I charge up my nervous energy to do so. If then a car suddenly appears, I instinctively jump out of its way. I then calm down and gradually unwind by continuing to cross the road when it is really safe or finding another place to cross. When I get home I may well talk to my partner about the fact that I nearly got knocked down by a car; here I am continuing to wind down by talking about it. Just before I go to sleep I may remember the incident again and finally let go of both the physiological and psychological remnants of the experience. This is a complete cycle.

However, in another example the cycle is not complete. Here, I am visiting an elderly relative and she says something that I strongly disagree with. I take a breath and move forwards in my chair to speak, but another relative talks and I decide that what I had to say was probably best kept to myself. However, by the time I get home I have got a headache and I feel frustrated and angry. In order to express and relax myself and complete the energetic cycle I might need to talk about the situation and express my frustration and anger in some way. The experience may also remind me of all the times in the past I did not speak out about what mattered to me, ie other incomplete cycles.

The biodynamic psychotherapist focuses energetically on her client and on her own responses to her client. You may be seated talking to each other, or you may be lying down on a mattress or couch. You will be supported to go into yourself, be with your experience of yourself right now and follow any impulse that you may be aware of. You let that impulse grow and develop. Your own impulse is followed, and the therapist holds and supports you to stay with this process. She does not impose an agenda of her own. Your impulse may lead you to experience a dilemma and the therapist will help you explore the mechanism by which you hold the energy of this dilemma in your body. For example, you might want to be close to the therapist or another person in your life, but feel acutely the decision that you made, perhaps at two years old, that you would not need anybody. The therapist's job is to help you stay with the blocked energy of this dilemma. This energy can then release, muscle contraction relaxes, and you can feel free of the dilemma.

Biodynamic massage

One aspect of biodynamic psychotherapy is biodynamic massage. This can either be a specialised form of massage on its own or part of biodynamic psychotherapy. In the latter the required training in psychotherapy must be completed. As a form of massage only, the therapist has usually completed less training than a biodynamic psychotherapist. As always it is important to know the qualification of the therapist.

The massage involves several different forms, such as basic touch, connective tissue massage (which can be for sedating or vitalising), holding, deep draining, working to redistribute the energy in the body or aura. Each of these particular forms has a range of strokes that are unique to this kind of massage.

Specific symptoms are seen as signs of an underlying imbalance and are not always considered to be the main focus. As with biodynamic psychotherapy, symptom reduction comes after the life force has been encouraged to flow more freely and the therapist does not attempt to cure or fix anything. Being with the client or patient without making any demands of her is the essence of this, and many other body therapies.

In biodynamic massage it is the peristaltic action in the gut (tummy rumblings) that the therapist uses as a guide to the emotional processes of the client. When we relax we slow our breathing and let go of muscle tensions. This is when these rumblings may be heard. The peristalsis may also happen at moments of significant change. Boyeson used a stethoscope to monitor the movements of the digestive tract and to guide the massage from moment to moment as the body responded to the touch.

This form of massage can be helpful for many conditions. It has been used with cardiac patients, Parkinson's disease, the elderly, acute admission patients in mental health, with the terminally ill and with those with learning difficulties. Gill Westland states, 'It could be applied in midwifery to neonates (newborns), preterm neonates, during labour and to labour companions. Nurses, occupational therapists, social workers, psychologists and doctors have used it in staff groups for stress management.'[9]

Gestalt

'Friend, don't be a perfectionist. Perfectionism is a curse and a strain. For you tremble lest you miss the bulls-eye. You are perfect if you let be... Friend, don't be afraid of mistakes. Mistakes are not sins. Mistakes are ways of doing something different, perhaps creatively new' (Fritz Perls, *In and Out the Garbage Pail*).[10]

Gestalt is a German word and there is no adequate English translation. It loosely means whole, configuration, integration, a unique patterning.

Fritz Perls is the 'grandfather' of gestalt therapy, which began in the 1940s as an exciting and innovative development of and reaction to psychoanalysis. He, like Reich, had been trained by Freud but also broke with the psychoanalytical tradition. He was influenced by five psychological and spiritual traditions: psychoanalysis, Reichian character analysis, existential philosophy, gestalt psychology and eastern religion. (Gestalt psychology was a theory of perception that developed in Germany. Perls then developed it into a therapy.)

Modern gestalt counselling/psychotherapy encompasses a broad and integrative theoretical base, which can be adapted to most people in many settings. The approach has a profound belief in the individual being responsible for the choices she makes in her own life, within the context of her environment. The one goal of gestalt therapy is awareness; 'to heighten the client's perception of her current function in relation to her environment, including aspects of her present ways of being which may be out of her awareness.'[11]

Instead of contacting repressed memories, gestalt therapy is a 'here and now' therapy. The focus is on the present tense so that a memory is viewed as an experience that is happening now and that has significance for the person right now, and can be brought to a conclusion so that it doesn't keep bothering them. Philosophically, this approach is described as phenomenological: what is, is; we are who we are; what we feel, we feel.

Perls discouraged his patients from interpreting, rationalising and intellectualising their lives. This is important, especially for some women who disparage themselves as non-intellectual. Interpretation and theory are strongly validated and in many ways overestimated in our culture, usually at the expense of actual moment-to-moment feeling.

We often avoid taking responsibility for ourselves and blame others for our situation. In addition we often project on to others that which really belongs to us. For example, we might imagine someone is angry with us, when in fact we are angry with them. Sheila Ernst and Lucy Goodison write, 'Gestalt therapy emphasises re-owning our projections and recognising our own power. Through gestalt people are encouraged to take responsibility for their own lives and to see that they do have the ability to take action in the present. This can be particularly helpful for women.'[12]

There are very real obstacles that block us from getting what we need in this society, and we often underestimate our own power to tackle those obstacles. By encouraging us to own our feelings, experiences and actions, gestalt therapy helps us to feel active rather than passive in our lives. For example, instead of using the word 'it', as in 'It feels a bit scary,' a gestalt therapist would encourage you to say 'I feel scared'. Using the word 'I' makes a difference in terms of taking responsibility for our thoughts, feelings and actions. Rather than look to why something is happening, we look to how we keep something happening. So this intervention could then lead to questions such as, 'How do you do that?' and 'What benefits does that give you?'

It is important to note that gestalt therapy itself has developed in all kinds of directions since Perls placed it on the map, and that Perls was quite an elderly man in the late 1960s when he became a kind of cult figure at Esalen in California. He has been criticised for not making the link between the personal and the political (unlike Reich). But Perls did reject the medical model that dominated psychotherapy. He stressed the inborn healthiness in everyone, with the belief that inside of us we do know what is best for us. Therapy is then a process of growing as we learn to listen more to the inner wisdom of our bodies. In this way, what might be considered neurotic can be redefined as actually the healthiest response we could make to a situation. For example, my night-terrors could be seen as the best way my organism knew to express my rage and fear, and to bring this into consciousness.

Gestalt therapy is based on awareness and the current reality of the client (phenomenology). Sometimes a gestalt therapist may suggest an experiment to her client. For example, the therapist may notice a repeated gesture, such as a clenched fist, or facial expression and bring this to the client's attention. If the client is willing to explore further then one way would be to ask her to speak as if from the clenched fist, as it may have something important to say that is outside the client's current awareness.

The gestalt therapist often supports the client to have dialogues based on present or past experiences, or based on fantasies of future experiences. This may be done internally, in the mind, with the client visualising aspects of themselves, or people they have relationships with; or it may be done through external creative activity such as drawing or painting. A commonly used gestalt technique involves using one or more empty chairs. The client imagines a part of herself, or another person, on the other chair (or chairs if more than one part or person is involved) and has a dialogue with them. This helps to externalise the internal dialogues that go on in our heads. This technique can also be used for rehearsing interviews, or a difficult conversation we need to have with someone. The therapist asks the client to visualise the other person or part of themselves in the empty chair and to speak to them. This is followed by switching chairs, and the client plays the person or the part responding. The dialogue continues with the client switching chairs, until her awareness of her projections is reached, or the conflict or 'unfinished business' is resolved.

Another useful technique is called the 'awareness continuum'. Here the therapist asks the client to bring her attention to what she is immediately aware of, by completing something called a sentence stem of 'I am aware of...'. There are three zones of awareness:

- inner: being everything inside my skin
- outer: being everything outside my skin that i can be aware of with my senses
- middle: being what I do with all this information in terms of thinking, fantasising.

An example would be: I feel my stomach is rumbling (inner); I hear the chimes of the ice-cream van (outer), and I imagine a double 99 ice-cream with two chocolate flakes (middle).

In respect of physicality, the gestalt therapist helps us become more aware of bodily sensations and the meanings behind particular symptoms. Here a symptom is perceived as an alienated part of ourself. As I have already indicated, a symptom often has a great deal to tell us, but we need to take time to pay attention to it and listen to the information it is giving us. Just as a symptom is sending messages to us, it is also expressing messages to those around us. Our symptoms can have a powerful effect on others.

Here is an example of dialoguing with a symptom and using VISUALISATION. Coral Burrows is in her early sixties. She works part-time as a medical secretary and has two adult children:

'I was getting migraine attacks every week, each lasting about two days. Allopathic medicine had little effect and, in any event, I did not wish to be taking drugs at such frequent intervals.

I had tried Chinese herbs, acupuncture, homoeopathy and biofeedback techniques without any appreciable improvement and it was while working with my therapist that I was gently introduced to visualisation. This was something I had always enjoyed as a relaxation aid but had not previously used in a focused way.

I began by concentrating on the migraine itself. I began to see it as a large, ugly black creature. It was blob shaped and had a malevolent expression and sharp claws. It was the claws that it dug into me that gave me the pain and tension on the right side of my head and that I could not shake off. I then drew it on a large sheet of paper. I used a lot of black crayon and I remember holding the crayon in my fist (as a child would) and pressing hard on the paper. In my next session I dialogued with the creature itself. I sat it on the chair opposite me and asked it what it wanted. "Control," it replied. "Why do you want to control me?" "Someone has to." "Why?" "Otherwise you'd just do as you wanted." "Would that matter?" It started to get agitated. "Of course it would. This way I'm in charge. You do what I tell you. You need me... I've been with you a long time." This stopped me talking to it – I didn't know how to reply. The harder I tried to push it away, the stronger it became, but I needed to disempower it.

"Okay," I said to it. "How can your controlling help me?" This seemed to throw it off course for a bit. "When you feel me in your shoulder and your head you know that I am warning you that things are getting difficult or too much for you to handle by yourself. You are feeling overwhelmed by events. The more you try to ignore me or to carry on, the tighter I have to hold on."

The above has made me take stock. I felt I had to be Super-woman and do everything myself. It has been very difficult for me to acknowledge that there are some things I find hard (I felt I should be able to do everything asked of me) and most of all *to ask for help*. I am still learning to listen to my inner voice but the migraines have stopped. If I think of the black blob now, I see it as on the same road as myself, but way back in the distance.'

Self-help
The above is called 'symptom dialoguing'. You can try this yourself:

Close your eyes and think of a physical symptom that is

bothering you; preferably one you can feel right now or, if not, one that bothers you quite often. See if you can recreate the feeling of the discomfort. Now focus your attention on this symptom with the intention of becoming more aware of the detail of it. Think about exactly what parts of your body are affected, and how you experience the different sensations. See if you can really accept this discomfort and let it into your awareness. See if you can increase this symptom, and notice how you do this, then do the opposite; see if you can reduce it by letting go in some way. Explore this in detail as much as possible.

The next step is that now you actually become this symptom. Feel yourself to be this symptom and ask yourself what you are like. What are your characteristics and attitudes and what do you do to this person (ie the rest of yourself)? Now, as the symptom, speak to the person and tell her what you do for her and how you make her feel.

Now become yourself again and speak back to the symptom. What do you say and how do you feel as you answer? Now continue the dialogue by switching back and forth between being the symptom and being yourself. As the symptom you can ask the person what you do for her, in what ways you are actually useful for her. You need to identify with whoever is doing the speaking at the time. When you have finished you need to sit quietly and absorb the experience. Then it is good to share it with someone, speaking in first-person present tense (as in 'I...'), or write it down in a journal.

An excellent book to explore the value of this kind of work is *Awareness* by John O Stevens. 'Whatever you find the symptom does for you, you might explore some means other than diseasing yourself that would achieve the same result. If you become ill in order to get a rest, perhaps you could be aware of your exhaustion, and take a rest before illness forces you to. If your symptom gets you care and attention from others, perhaps there is some other way that you could ask for this care and attention'.[13]

Rebirthing (or conscious connected breathing)

'Simply breathing – simply choosing to breathe, now, with conscious, creative awareness – can be the resolution of all that has come before and the evolution of all to follow'.[14]

Rebirthing utilises a defined breathing technique called 'conscious connected breathing' to bring about a detailed awareness of your own mind, body and emotions. This kind of breathing is learning to breathe in a circular way with no pause between inhaling and exhaling and no holding of air. Breathing out should be without effort and breathing in involves a willingness to open up and receive. It is about being in the present and surrendering to what actually is, rather than what you think could or should be. It is the art of not holding your breath.

Rebirthing has a number of important basic premises: it is about appreciating the miracle of existence; of acknowledging that we are fundamentally innocent when we come into this world; that people choose to interpret and experience in the way that they do; that at any given time we are doing the best we can (later we increase our consciousness and perhaps would choose differently); that we each have a personal lie (that is, that deep down we tell ourselves something, such as 'I am unlovable', or 'I am not wanted' or 'I am not good enough', or 'I am weak'). We then build psychological defences from that place. As a response we may overcompensate by becoming a high achiever, or we may try to blot out the pain by repeated addictive behaviour (eg alcohol, drugs or sex).

Rebirthing was founded in California by Leonard Orr in the mid-1970s. He described the therapy not in terms of teaching a person to breathe but rather as the intuitive and gentle learning of breathing from the breath itself. Rebirthing enables the body-mind to restructure itself in a way that potentially increases happiness, effectiveness and good health. The rebirthing practitioner, who will have cleared her own birth trauma and be ready to assist others, will support her client to go only as deeply into herself as she feels safe to do.

Leonard Orr also researched breathing with 'wet rebirthing', which takes place with the person being in warm water. The idea of this was to stimulate felt memories of being in the womb.

Breath is the means by which we sustain aliveness in our bodies and either increase our experience of safety and pleasure or reinforce our feelings of suffering and pain. Physiologically, the breath is a limitless source of vitality and aliveness that is always available to us. The quality of breathing affects blood oxygenation, essential for building and maintaining healthy tissue. It also has a primary role in releasing chemical toxins and waste, thus cleansing and purifying our bodily systems. If the body is gradually polluted because we are not breathing properly, we are not getting rid of toxins and wastes as quickly as we are taking them in. Disease is therefore likely to ensue. Practitioner of rebirthing, Bernadette Riley, also tells us, 'Frequently, the strategies for coping with uncomfortable feelings are aimed at trying to avoid what is going on. A favourite way we do this is to hold our breath. When we hold our breath we lose our awareness, suppress our feelings and start reacting rather than responding... we block off any creative solution to the problem.'[15]

This releasing of old memories is very powerful. Gunnel Minnet states, 'Before the brain is fully developed, memories were recorded and stored as bodily sensations in various parts of the body. It is not possible to reach this type of memory through the mind. These early memories have not left a sufficient imprint in the brain, only in the area of the body which was involved in the original experience'.[16]

Rebirthing asserts that thought is creative. A rebirther shows her client how to work with positive affirmations (see Chapter 2). The 'personal lie' mentioned earlier is a negative affirmation. However, the rebirther supports you to acknowledge the negative messages, not suppress them.

Rebirthing can be done individually, with a practitioner or in a group. Individual sessions take approximately two hours, and you lie on a mattress on the floor, or on a treatment couch. Your practitioner guides you and may direct changes in the pace and style of your breathing if it seems that this would help to release tensions trapped in muscles and other parts of your body. Her task is to help you discover your own rhythm.

When you feel safe enough to let go completely there can be a spontaneous memory of the first breath ever taken. This can be a very deep spiritual experience, with feelings of joy and pleasure in being alive. Anna Bondizio writes, 'Many people experienced trauma of some kind before, during or after birth. They may have struggled through the birth canal, or been forced out by forceps that scrunched and twisted the head. They may have come out breech or have shared their mother's anaesthetic in the process. Emotionally they may have experienced terror, fear or loneliness ... Many felt unloved or rejected for being the wrong sex according to the expectations of the parents ... A frequent experience was receiving a good smack to get the breath going'.[17]

Benefits

The potential benefits of rebirthing are many. Although the methods vary, these benefits are shared with the other body psychotherapies in this chapter:

- it can encourage you to uncover and challenge limiting beliefs and thoughts
- you can gain new ideas and insights
- you can discover new capabilities you were unaware of
- you can experience greater self-empowerment and find hidden strengths
- it can help you be more open about yourself and be able to communicate this
- you can feel more in touch with your needs as they arise, as your muscles relax and become more sensitive
- you can develop a greater sense of trust in yourself, your relationships and the universe
- you can connect with your inner spiritual awareness, and this can lead to changes of perception of unwanted situations.

Carolyn, a social worker in her fifties, has been involved with rebirthing for many years. She says:

'Of course, each rebirthing session is experienced differently for each person, so no two sessions are ever alike, and you cannot predict what might happen. You need to trust your own body-mind to know what needs healing next. Not everyone re-experiences birth or even early childhood memories, but the technique is still justified in my experience.'

And fifty-year-old Bernadette Riley, quoted earlier, who is now a trained practitioner of rebirthing herself, describes her first rebirthing experience:

'My first rebirthing experience was physically very uncomfortable to begin with. There were all sorts of strange tightening sensations and I wanted it to stop. My rebirther encouraged me to have a little willingness to be with this discomfort. Then I began to feel as if I was *being breathed* and the breathing became effortless. The discomfort in my body vanished and I felt euphoric. Pictures of my parents flashed through my mind. They were younger and were watching over me and in one exquisite moment I realised I had parcelled away somewhere in my body an angry belief that I was unlovable, and that I had to keep it hidden in case I might be ignored and isolated. It was an extraordinary and beautiful experience to realise that they were and are loving human beings doing their best for me. As I went through more rebirthing sessions my eyes opened to unconscious habits. I discovered that I could begin to make many more conscious choices by being in contact with my experience of the here and now and with my potential.'

Rebirthing practitioners themselves are experienced and trained professionals who, because of their own sense of safety, integrity and compassion, can guide people through rebirthing sessions. As with other forms of therapy it is essential that the practitioner is well trained and therefore knows what she is doing.

Self-help

Twenty Connected Breaths: this means connecting the 'in' breath with the 'out' breath and the 'out' breath with the 'in' breath. Take the breaths in and out through your nose. This exercise is adapted from the founder of rebirthing, Leonard Orr. It only takes thirty seconds to do this and it will bring fresh life energy into your mind and body:

1. Take four short breaths.
2. Take one big breath.
3. Do four sets of five breaths: that is, four sets of four short breaths plus one long breath without stopping, for a total of twenty breaths.

Hypnotherapy

The main theory behind therapeutic hypnotherapy is that most problems, including many physical ones, have their origins in subconscious patterns. Subconscious means under or behind. The subconscious part of the mind is always present and aware.

Hypnosis is a natural state of mind. Under ordinary everyday circumstances we go into hypnosis spontaneously, normally and naturally. If we have been told over and over that we are very good or no good at something, we come to believe it totally and fall in to some kind of trance. Other forms of hypnosis are:

- day dreaming
- just before we fall asleep
- as we are coming out of sleep, but before being awake
- whenever we are completely *in* a feeling such as laughter, anger, fear, crying etc
- whenever we are shocked by something, eg an event, good or bad news and so on.

In these situations we instinctively alter our state to deal with ourselves. Susan Wilmott, a practising hypnotherapist, tells us, 'The hypnotherapist and client use this natural state quite purposefully and with intent, which is really the only thing that makes it different from what we're constantly engaged with otherwise.' Stephen Fulder describes hypnosis as a state in which '(a) the cognitive controls over the mind are loosened or dissociated; and (b) the person is not asleep and can receive and act on messages.'[18]

Hypnosis has been used for therapeutic purposes since ancient times. Egyptian priests used incense with incantations to induce hypnotic states for healing. In tribal societies, shamans, medicine men and witch-doctors create hypnotic trances for rituals and healing. Some of the roots of modern hypnotherapy are shared with those of SPIRITUAL HEALING (see Chapter 8), such as the work of Franz Anton Mesmer. He was a charismatic therapist in the eighteenth century, who treated large numbers of people successfully by inducing deep trances. His system was called 'animal magnetism' and he believed that the human body had a magnetic polarity that was surrounded by a force field. Unfortunately he roused a lot of antagonism, since scientists rejected his methods and the Church viewed his work as a mystical heresy because he believed it came from the universe, not from the person. The actual word neuro-hypnosis, meaning sleep of the nervous system, was coined in 1841 by James Braid, a Scottish doctor.

The modern hypnotherapist attempts to alter ingrained patterns of behaviour. As already said, and contrary to what a lot of people think, hypnotherapy does not involve going into a sleep state. However, it does involve the client becoming very relaxed so that the therapist can work with her on a deep level. This altered state of consciousness is often called trance or hypnosis. To support the client entering the hypnotic trance the therapist speaks in a way that slows; a relaxing, controlled and confident way. This allows the client to effect a detached and concentrated state. One common method of induction is the therapist counting the client down from ten to one. Another method is to use gentle music to help with the relaxation process. Relaxation therapy and CREATIVE VISUALISATION are other ways to describe hypnosis.

As with all therapies, it is important that there is support between therapist and client. The process may take a few minutes or longer. The depth of trance is determined by the client, not the therapist, and this depth has no correlating effect on outcome. In fact a renowned hypnotherapist, Milton Erikson, developed a method of hypnosis that was so subtle it seemed as if he and the patient were having a normal conversation. Erikson observed how normal the hypnotic state is and used it positively.

It was not until the 1950s that medical doctors began to shift their disbelief that the mind could influence organic diseases. What used to be termed psychosomatic conditions and deemed unimportant have more recently come to be seen as significant, showing us that the mind has in fact considerable influence in health or illness. A British Medical Association committee eventually approved hypnotherapy for certain medical conditions and behavioural problems.[19]

The process of hypnotherapy might include giving the subconscious mind or 'out of consciousness' mind positive suggestions or suggestions that help the person to sort through inner conflicts. Repetition is often used. The effectiveness of hypnosis as a therapy does not just depend on the extent to which a person is able to retain a suggestion in her waking state. Some clients completely forget in the wide awake state, and still notice changes.

Autohypnosis (self-hypnosis) is where the therapist trains the patient to hypnotise herself. This means she can continually reinforce the therapist's suggestions. This can be invaluable for pain relief. Obviously using your subconscious mind to bypass your conscious mind is something of a challenge. You need to be in a state of relaxed uncritical awareness — the 'hypnoidal' state — in order to do this. Sometimes we are unable to stop critical voices in the mind. Fortunately this makes no difference to the subconscious mind; it can still shift despite these critical messages. Self-hypnosis is easily learned by recognising it.

Benefits
Hypnotherapy is useful for:

* curing obsessive habits, especially smoking
* allergies
* asthma

- anxiety and panic attacks
- insomnia
- menstrual disorders
- infertility
- ovarian cysts
- migraine and tension headaches
- tinnitus
- chronic pain
- eczema and psoriasis.

Because hypnotherapy supports the person to be in a particular mental state it is being used to help people in the final stages of terminal illness. It not only reduces symptoms, it helps relieve anxiety and fear. Self-hypnosis has been used during labour, to help the mother relax, reduce pain, reduce or even eliminate use of medication, and thus help keep both the mother and baby alert. For decades it has been used in cases of Caesarean section when the mother has been allergic to anaesthetic.

Contraindications

A hypnotherapy session usually begins with a complete medical history to determine if there are any contra-indications, such as a serious heart condition, or if another therapy would be more appropriate. Although this therapy is very safe, an area of risk could be manipulation by the hypnotist. Clearly hypnotherapists need training in psycho-therapy and to work to high ethical standards. This is where knowing the difference between hypnotists who are stage performers and clinical hypnotherapists is extremely important.

Chapter Ten

Energy Movement Systems

Healing ourselves through moving is natural. Moving helps to release old, stored-up and unexpressed feelings, leaving us to feel more free to be authentic in each moment.

Some of the most common systems have been included. These forms of bodywork often, although not always, involve the individual learning of specific sequences of movements and positions. They must be learned properly to be safe and effective. Always choose a well-qualified teacher. Many of these systems come from the East and have existed for centuries.

Yoga

Yoga is a complete science of life that began in India many thousands of years ago and nowadays there are many schools with differing approaches. The oldest archaeological evidence of the existence of yoga is a number of stone seals showing figures in yogic postures. These were excavated from the Indus Valley and are thought to date from around 3000 BC. Yoga is first mentioned in the vast collection of scriptures called the Vedas, some of which date from 2500 BC. The Upanishads, forming the later part of the Vedas, provide the main foundation of yoga teaching and of the philosophy known as Vedanta. The idea that is central to Vedanta is that underlying the entire universe is one absolute reality or consciousness, known as Brahman.

Perhaps the best known yogic scriptures are the *Bhagavadgita*, written by Vyasa around the sixth century BC, and the Yogasutras, written by Patanjali. 'The soul that moves in the world of the senses and yet keeps the sense in harmony... finds rest in quietness' (*Bhagavadgita*). The purpose of the different aspects of practising yoga is to reunite the individual self (jiva) with the Absolute or pure consciousness (Brahman). The word yoga actually means 'joining'. 'Union with this unchanging reality liberates the spirit from all sense of separation, freeing it from the illusion of time, space and causation. It is only our own ignorance, our inability to discriminate between the real and unreal, that prevents us from realising our true natures.'[1] Little is known of the author of the Yogasutras, other than that he was called Patanjali and lived around the second century BC. Alternatively there are those who believe the author is the incarnation of Ananta, the divine serpent that supports the world.

The inspiration for the Yogasutras is more certain. This came from the Vedas: a collection of six schools of Indian thought that inspired the sages of old. The Vedas inspired all the major Indian texts.

Words of each sutra put together do not even form a sentence. The style is terse and condensed to allow for the oral tradition of teaching. Patanjali's definition of yoga is: 'Yoga is the ability to direct the mind exclusively towards an object and sustain that direction without any distraction.'[2] Translated by Desikachar, Patanjali's book is dedicated to this ideal, with ways and means to achieve this carefully explained. He refers to the eight limbs of yoga.[3] These are:

1. Yama: our relationship to the world in which we live
2. Niyama: our relationship to ourselves

3. Asana: to work on the body through specific postures
4. Pranayama: to work on the breath through breath control
5. Pratyahara: to control our senses
6. Dharana: to learn to focus our minds
7. Dhyana: to focus more deeply on the object of our concentration
8. Samadhi: to integrate totally with the object of our concentration.

The ancient yogis perceived the physical body as a vehicle, the driver being the mind, the true identity being the soul. Action, emotion and intelligence are the three forces that pull the body-vehicle. Our health and development depends on these three forces being in balance.

Styles of yoga
There are several different kinds of yoga. Hatha yoga is a general term used in the West and within this there are different branches of yoga that focus on slightly different aspects of physical and mental exercise. Here are a few of the main ones:

Ashtanga yoga at present is very fashionable among some film stars, most notably Madonna. It is a dynamic, fast-paced version of yoga in which the postures and breathing techniques are continuous. Heat is generated and this purifies the body and makes it more flexible. There is also meditation at the end of a class to relax the mind. Because of the sustained movement, often for an hour and a half, it builds up muscle tone. It is of interest to people who like gymnastics and have a strong body. On an emotional level it can challenge feelings such as fear.

Iyengar yoga is more static with an emphasis on precise, exact posture. For instance, one asana may be practised for several minutes. The postures are adapted according to your ability and range of movement. The benefits include the development of mental and physical awareness, a decongested and rested body, and improvements to respiration, muscle tone, heart and lung function, greater stamina and emotional calming.

Sivananda yoga focuses more on breathing and meditation. This includes chanting mantras (the repetition of one sound such as 'om') to focus attention. This is a very gentle style and good for people whose body does not respond well to dynamic activity. It is suitable for people of all ages. As with other styles benefits include improved flexibility, greater energy and a strengthened immune system. Emotionally it helps clear the mind and lift your spirits.

Viniyoga yoga is the style that I personally practise. Viniyoga adapts to individual needs, integrating movement, breathing and mental focus for better physical and mental health as well as spiritual awareness. It is relevant to the person and the situation. The precise use of the breath particularly during postures is a powerful tool to influence a person's mental and physical well-being, clarity and insight. This approach involves one to one lessons, which I find valuable because of my history of back pain. Your teacher creates a programme adapted to your own specific needs, and your relationship with her is valued. Small group classes are available for those without especially limiting problems, who prefer working in a group. This form of yoga shares the major benefits with those already mentioned.

The physiology of yoga
According to yogic philosophy aging is largely an artificial condition, caused mostly by poisoning ourselves through the food we eat, lack of exercise, pollution, stress and lack of quietness. We can reduce the catabolic process of cell

deterioration through keeping the body parts clean and well lubricated. Although many of us practise yoga for specific physical conditions such as improving breathing and posture, whole body stretching and muscle toning, it is much more than physical exercise. With meditation and good nutrition it is a whole way of life. Yoga exercises – or 'asanas' as they are called – use every part of the body, stretching and toning the muscles and joints, the spine and entire skeletal system. Not only do they work on the frame of the body but also on its internal organs, glands and nerves. There are special asanas for pregnancy.

Benefits

As already indicated under the section on yoga styles, the benefits of practising yoga regularly are extremely wide reaching. The yogic breathing exercises, 'pranayama', revitalise the body and help mind-control. They also work on the chakra energy systems of the body (see Chapter 8). Like the hands-on therapies, yoga can help you respect and like your body whatever shape or size you are. For maximum benefit yoga needs to be a daily practice. However, if you are basically well you will definitely benefit from a regular weekly class, and twice a week is even better. Here are some more general benefits, many of which have been proved by medical research. Regular practice can help with:

- relief of high blood pressure
- arthritis
- chronic fatigue
- asthma
- heart conditions
- tension and backache.

Involuntary functions such as temperature, heartbeat and blood pressure have been shown in laboratory tests to confirm that the serious practitioner of yoga can develop the ability to consciously control these functions.

'One study of the effects of Hatha yoga over six months demonstrated the following effects: significantly increased lung capacity and respiration; reduced body weight and girth; an improved ability to resist stress; and a decrease in cholesterol and blood sugar level – all resulting in a stabilising and restorative effect on the body's natural systems.'[4] Although it will not necessarily cure a chronic condition, it can improve quality of life considerably. People with ME can stimulate energy by doing gentle movements and breathing and so combat fatigue. It is definitely a way of keeping our bodies fit and supple.

Contraindications
You must learn yoga techniques from a fully qualified and experienced yoga teacher, as many asanas are dangerous if you are suffering from spinal injuries or heart disease or high blood pressure. Some asanas are not suitable if you are pregnant or if you have your period. Before practising allow at least two hours after a meal, and half an hour after a snack.

Lou's story illustrates how yoga can help with serious problems. Please note that she sees a yoga teacher on a one-to-one basis. If you do have a serious condition, going along to a general yoga class once a week may not be a good idea. If you do, you must speak to the teacher and have her monitor your movements.

'I am forty-six years old – married with two children aged twenty-seven and sixteen...I discovered about four years ago that a childhood injury had left me with damaged vertebrae in my neck. This damage forced the C5/6 disc into the cord. This was removed and a metal fusion put in. Then the disc at 6/7 slipped and has since fused on its own.

I have damage in the spinal cord, which causes muscle

fatigue and pain, mainly in my shoulders, hands, arms and legs. My bladder is a bit of an enigma, and I get the odd bit of twitching and rashes.

I had started yoga classes about twelve years ago. I was also having counselling and the two things went together quite well. Yoga has helped in many ways. By being aware of my body I can help myself by improving posture, and ease out aching muscles with yoga exercises. I can also use relaxation, breathing, self-healing and visualisation techniques to help and empower myself to take control of my body's health. The cord damage came as a shock and yoga has helped me keep a confident and positive attitude. I have a personal yoga teacher, who has experience of remedial yoga.

My osteopath diagnosed spinal cord injury first. I went to see her after fruitless visits to the GP about pain in my knees and pins and needles in my hands. I have been treated at least every two weeks for the past three years. I feel the cranial osteopathy has been really helpful, encouraging the flow of fluid in the spinal cord and as I tend to pull muscles very easily it's a great help to have my body realigned regularly.

Both my osteopath and yoga teacher are women. I am not sure I would have had such a good working relationship with them if they were men. They both emphasise my responsibility and ability to help myself and encourage me when I'm in a down patch. I would recommend osteopathy and yoga to anyone and everyone. Of course the teacher/practitioner should be qualified. Yoga classes vary hugely. You have to choose the right one for your needs ...

Self-help techniques for pain, relaxation (yoga) and the visualisations for self-healing are simple. My own favourite is after a relaxation exercise to see myself walking along the cliffs and going into a healing space – a cave or wood or waterfall – and spend time there taking in a healing elixir, then cheerfully walking back...'

Marilyn Kirby, who has also suffered from back pain for twenty years, writes:

'My most recent therapy has been the one with which I noticed almost immediate results, and that is yoga. In just three weeks I have noticed considerable difference in my ability to move freely and bend. I no longer feel stiff and suffer joint aches when I wake in the morning. The teacher incorporates the spiritual element of yoga, which is important to me. I feel as if my energy levels are higher now that I practise yoga every day.'

Self-help

Both asana and pranayama practice is more beneficial when taught by a competent yoga teacher. This is even more important if you have chronic physical or psychological problems.

The first requirement for pranayama practice is to sit comfortably with your back straight, but not rigid, in a cross-legged seated position if you are healthy and strong. If, for example, you have heart or low-energy problems you may benefit from sitting on a chair. You should be alert but without tension.

Observation is the second requirement for pranayama practice. Be aware of the body and mind response to your breathing. As with the asana practice allow your breathing capacity to develop slowly, without pushing beyond your comfortable limit. There are many different breathing techniques, each one of therapeutic value. However, for a safe, simple technique to experience the breath, observe and feel the movement in your chest on the inhale and the abdomen on the exhale. If you practise this technique daily you should soon be aware of the potential of the breath to calm and relax your mind on one level, but also to sharpen and improve your concentration.

A simple physical self-help movement, helping combine your breathing with movement, is to stand or sit (again upright but not rigid) and as you breathe in raise your arms to the side. Note that both the movement and your breathing needs to be as slow as possible. On the out breath you lower your arms. Repeat this a few times, maintaining the slowness and the breath and movement coordination.

Tai chi

There are a variety of styles of tai chi, which originate from different families (such as the Yang style or the Wu style). The more martial art forms of tai chi are referred to as tai chi ch'uan. Ch'uan means 'the supreme ultimate fist'. Tai chi itself is more to do with the development of vital energy (chi) than with fighting techniques. It is not competitive.

There is a story that a thirteenth-century Taoist monk, Chang San-feng, invented the movements because he had been watching a crane and a snake fighting and was struck by how softness and yielding combined so effectively in this combative situation. Although it was once a secret art, tai chi is now practised for health, meditation, enjoyment and self-defence by millions of people in China and around the world.

The different styles of tai chi involve series of postures each called a form. These are performed in a slow, continuous sequence. The focus of these fluent movements is on the dan tien (or hara)[5] and the weight is brought down into the lower half of the body. From here the person is 'centred' and chi can move freely.

The movements reflect the Taoist philosophy of harmony with nature, for example, you learn to be rooted like a tree, with your full weight resting on the ground; the waist is flexible, like clouds waving across the open sky; the mind is still and calm, large like a mountain; and the spirit is allowed to soar, as though a graceful heron had just spread its wings.

In China it is prescribed by doctors in conjunction with other treatments. Because it is gentle it is suitable for the elderly, the very young and the physically weak. In China people practise tai chi in parks at dawn. In Chinese philosophy, nature's chi flows at its strongest at sunrise.

Benefits

The benefits of regular practice of tai chi are extensive:

- increased muscle tone, which improves circulation of the blood and lymph systems
- opening of joints, especially the knees, leading to help with arthritis and rheumatism
- strengthening of the lower back
- massaging of the internal organs
- strengthening of the intestines and help with elimination
- can help with ulcers and nervous disorders through the calming effect
- improved heart function because the breathing deepens, the blood and brain get more oxygen, and the blood vessels can become more open and flexible
- promotion of concentration, confidence, self-control, serenity and awareness.

Tai chi is good for elderly people for it has a reputation for increasing health and promoting longevity. Because the body's energy flow is increased, with regular practice the immune system is boosted and so sickness can be prevented.

Tai chi may also improve circulation of the cerebrospinal fluid. Regular practice improves coordination and balance, making it especially useful for the elderly, stroke victims and people with Parkinson's disease. Studies and anecdotal evidence suggest that, with regular practice, it may also help with asthma and other lung/breathing problems, multiple sclerosis, ME and ankylosing spondilosis.

The theory of YIN and YANG, the law of complementary polarities, is intrinsic to tai chi (see Chapter 7). 'Active relaxation' is an example of this. The movements of tai chi turn the body on a centre line from the top of the head down to the feet, so that one half of the body moves to the right and the other to the left with this centre line remaining perfectly still. Even the name tai chi ch'uan contains the yin/yang idea. Elaine Stillerman describes this: 'The "supreme ultimate fist" actually purports a principle of softness...outer suppleness and inner stability can overcome violent movements, like a blade of grass yielding to the wind.'[6] Nothing is forced, it is the art of non-exertion. We are accustomed to dealing with the world with effort and struggle. Instead of pushing, in tai chi you use movements in the form of retreats which bring a yielding and a feeling of softness. By moving very slowly the body's habitual responses are bypassed.

Tai chi is taught in classes, although the practice is done on a regular basis at home by oneself. Dianne Spencer, a tai chi instructor, says, 'While it can be nice to do a set on your own I always get more out of it when I practise with others; it seems to magnify the energy somehow.'

Betty Puleston is forty-four years old and has a history of knee problems, ME[7] and Raynaud's disease.[8] Here is her story:

'I used to do a lot of sport when I was younger, but when I was eighteen or nineteen I started getting a lot of pain in my left knee. The problem worsened until, in my early twenties, I had to have major surgery. The pain persisted and I have since had two more operations on the knee; one in 1993 to repair the disc cartilage, and another in 1997 to remove crumbling cartilage. I've also had a cartilage repair operation on the right knee. But that's not my only problem.

In 1987 I had a bout of flu. I had just started a new job and didn't want to take any time off, so I kept going. Eventually, though, I couldn't drag myself out of bed. I spent six months virtually housebound. I could hardly walk but, if I used a wheelchair, I suffered awful dizziness. My memory was terrible and I was so weak I had to ask my neighbour to plait my daughter's hair for me.

It was a relief to discover, in 1988, that I had ME – even though I was told there wasn't really any treatment. By then I was suffering bad back pain and had also developed Raynaud's disease. To compound things, in 1989 my husband walked out on me, so I had a lot of emotional stress to deal with, and in 1990 I broke my elbow very badly, which led to severe shoulder pain.

Then, in 1993, a friend of mine who had MS told me she had started learning tai chi through the Taoist Tai Chi Society of Great Britain. She said she was sure it was improving her balance and I decided that if she could do it, so could I. To start with, I couldn't manage to do the full two-hour class standing up. And when I got home I found I couldn't practise much because I couldn't remember what I had just been taught. That said, I found I was sleeping better and, before I got to the end of the beginners' class, I realised that, for the first time in ages, I was able to get into bed and lie flat out straight away. Before that, I had had to lie on my side until my back relaxed sufficiently for me to be able to straighten out.

I started attending a second beginners' class, which helped reinforce the moves in my memory, and suddenly I discovered that my balance had improved to the extent that I could stand on one leg to do the kick moves. From there, I seemed to go from strength to strength.

It wasn't all easy though. In 1994 I had to have my gall bladder removed, and then I discovered I was pregnant. I developed pregnancy diabetes and had to have my son by

Caesarean section a month early but, compared with my other pregnancies, this one was easy. With both my daughters I had had to go into hospital weeks before the birth because I was in so much pain with back problems, but with Josh, I was doing tai chi right up to two weeks before the birth.

My circulation has improved, too, so the Raynaud's has eased a bit, and tai chi also seems to have helped me emotionally; partly I think because of the support I receive from other members of the society, but also because it helps calm me down.

Today I'm still registered disabled. I can't work and I'm in pain all the time with my knee. But my back and shoulder are a lot better and the ME has improved considerably. It's strange, but I can do tai chi all day – I've been on five- and seven-day workshops, and I'm an instructor myself now – but I still can't walk very far. How it works is a bit of a mystery, but the point is, when I'm doing tai chi, I feel normal.'

Chi gung

This is also a total exercise and meditation system (sometimes spelt 'qigong') that is a part of CHINESE MEDICINE and is thousands of years old. It works on the ACUPUNCTURE meridians running through the body and through which energy (chi) flows. Just as with acupuncture, any illness, disease or mental or physical problem is viewed as the result of blockage or imbalance of energy in the meridians. Doing chi gung breathing or physical exercises helps to unblock, balance and promote the healthy flow of chi throughout the body.

Chi gung combines breathing techniques and mental concentration with precise movements and stationary positions. The focus is on having your attention on the movement, breathing or positions so as to be with it moment by moment in an easy way. There are single movement exercises and series of movements that make up short chi gung forms. The movements are gentle, precise and often elegant. Some forms also utilise imagery, such as visualising specific organs, and releasing into free movement.

As with other movement systems, in chi gung the use of the breath is key to its benefits. It postulates that deep breathing can gradually cleanse the body of pollutants and improve lung capacity. This in turn creates more energy. In her book *Supertherapies*, Jane Alexander states that in China people with tuberculosis have been cured solely with the use of chi gung, and that the average person breathes around sixteen times a minute while someone who regularly practises chi gung breathes slowly and deeply just five or six times.

People find chi gung enjoyable and helpful just with ten to twenty minutes practice a day, or alternatively with attending a weekly chi gung class. It is advisable to learn the exercises with a chi gung practitioner. There are individual and group classes. Once you've learned the exercises, you can do them on your own. Alternatively you can continue in a weekly class if you would like that support or think you won't be able to find time to do the exercises on your own.

Anyone, including disabled people, can do chi gung because a lot of the movements are slow, do not require a lot of physical strength and can be adapted to individual physical limitations. It can be beneficial in pregnancy and for the labour, birth and the newborn. However, it is very important to do this in consultation with a chi gung practitioner, and to follow your deep sense of how much (if any) and what kind of chi gung would be helpful to you at this time.

If you would like to use chi gung to help with a specific illness, contact a practitioner to see what the best approach may be. Some acupuncturists are also chi gung practitioners and combine the two disciplines as one healing process.

The exercises are a powerful tool for energetic self-help,

which can be used in conjunction with other forms of complementary medicine, including Chinese herbs. There are no contraindications as long as you tell your tutor or practitioner about any medical problems you may have.

Pilates

Pilates is a conditioning technique that tones the muscles and improves posture and flexibility safely throughout the whole body. It concentrates on strengthening muscles without forcing them, using slow and controlled movements to avoid injury.

Pilates, named after Joseph Pilates (born in Germany in 1880), was originally described as a contrology. Joseph Pilates had been a sickly child who overcame his physical weakness by becoming a keen sportsman. He devised a fitness programme during the First World War when he was in England and interned because of his nationality. The story goes that he claimed it was because of his regime that not one of his fellow internees died from the influenza epidemic that killed thousands of people in 1918. After the war he came into the world of dance. His methods were adopted by both ballet companies and institutions such as police forces. Living in New York, top dancers, actors, athletes and the rich and famous were attracted to a physical exercise programme that 'built strength without adding bulk, balancing that strength with flexibility, and achieving the perfect harmony between mind and muscle.'[9] There are now more than five hundred studios in the US.

It was Alan Herdman who first brought the Pilates method to the UK, where he set up a studio in central London. Here, in around 1975, dancer and actor Gordon Thomson trained to teach the method.

Lynne Robinson is one woman behind the growth in popularity of this form of bodywork. Lynne had suffered years of back trouble: 'She had virtually given up hope of being free from back and neck pain and any sort of exercise – even gentle yoga – aggravated the situation.'[10] She was helped by Pilates teacher Penny Lately and Penny's osteopath husband Philip, and now has a back that is completely reshaped.

There are many varieties of Pilates being taught, because the essence of the teaching is that the technique is adapted to suit the individual. This means that new exercises are developed and special equipment designed to overcome injuries and postural problems. Pilates' 'disciples' went on to teach their own versions of his methods. I like this idea of a method being able to absorb new ideas and grow organically, rather than be fixed to a set of rules.

The difference between these exercises and keep-fit or stretch and tone exercises is that no movement is made without correct postural alignment being taken into consideration. There are six basic principles, plus two that have been added, that underpin all the exercises:

1. concentration
2. breathing
3. placement
4. centring
5. control
6. flowing movement, plus
7. relaxation
8. stamina.

Benefits

This method of bodywork is particularly good for:

- sports persons who have been injured; sports performers such as skaters and horse jumpers where postural alignment is important
- performers such as dancers, actors and musicians, where

good posture is essential; chronic back pain sufferers whose problems come from postural problems
- first-time exercisers or those getting back into exercise after a break
- sufferers of repetitive strain injury
- older people who want to maintain their mobility and independence
- people suffering from stress and stress-related illnesses.

Pilates teachers always suggest that it is important to consult your doctor before embarking on a new fitness regime if you have chronic muscular skeletal problems.

Contraindications

Jan Morley, aged thirty-seven, is a designer. Here is her experience:

'Pilates is very gentle to start off with and then you learn that every exercise that you do, you can choose to do harder. It's all about strengthening your muscles, especially your pelvis. I went because my back muscles were always very tight. My osteopath also suggested I go because of my posture; I wasn't standing properly and this was affecting my legs, causing tense muscles, which affected my whole body. The exercises have loosened up my back muscles. I feel so much better. My back and my knees have stopped hurting. Pilates re-educates your muscles so you can hold yourself in your correct posture. It tones you up wonderfully.'

Feldenkrais

'Feldenkrais invites you to learn how to move in a new way... This could include learning how to sit at a computer and not get back pain, relearn how to move after a stroke, or give a presentation and develop a body rapport with the audience.'[11]

This method improves freedom of movement and flexibility. It is about learning body awareness through sensory experience, and being with the process of movement; how it is formed, and what its potential may be. It is concerned with function rather than posture, and how we can function with ease and grace, using less effort and less limitation. Someone trained in Feldenkrais becomes an astute observer of the movement of themselves and others.

Moshe Feldenkrais, who was born in the Ukraine in 1904 and died in 1984, applied his background in physics and engineering to the study of human movement because he had chronic knee problems caused by an old soccer injury. He discovered that, just as the brain tells the body what to do, so the body can also instruct the brain by demonstrating the easiest, most effective ways to move. What then happens is a reprogramming of the brain. One main principle of this method is based on the idea that 'the less effort you make, the more sensitive you will become'.

As Chantal Kickz explains, 'If I carry a fridge on my back, half a pound of sugar can be added and I won't feel the difference. But if I'm holding a feather between my fingers and a bee comes to sit on it, even if my eyes are closed, I will feel the difference.'[12] The message here is that the less muscular effort we make, then the freer our nervous system is to feel and become aware. Feldenkrais teacher Scott Clark describes his work: 'We offer our students clear alternatives in movement, then let their natural sense of ease and power make the choices. If the alternatives are clear in sensation, not just ideas or concepts, it works. The process is sometimes like a set of physical riddles, partially designed so that the sensory message drops home before the intellect has a chance to grab it and interfere.'

Feldenkrais bodywork comes in two forms: individual hands-on sessions called Functional Integration and movement re-education classes called Awareness Through Movement. Functional Integration is a series of gentle manipulations to improve breathing and alignment. Feldenkrais calls this 'showing the body how to move with functional intelligence'. Neshama Franklin, in *The New Holistic Health Handbook*, writes, 'But it's more than physical manipulation. After a session I emerged with one shoulder perceptibly lower than the other. I expressed concern that I might have become permanently out of whack, but the practitioner...assured me that if my body liked how the lowered shoulder felt, the higher one would gradually drop to the same level. Within a few days, it happened, and my shoulders felt more relaxed than they had in years.'[13]

The Awareness Through Movement is done in classes, so it is less expensive than individual sessions. Here you are taught a series of gentle non-aerobic motions with the key aim being bodily and sensory awareness. You learn to scan your body to find tense areas, and to compare differences between your limbs. You are guided verbally to move gently and slowly. Most of the time you will be lying on the floor, sometimes sitting or standing. You may focus on one particular function, such as lifting the head.

My own experience of Feldenkrais some years ago has stayed in my memory. I remember feeling much lighter after the classes and certainly much more aware of how I was moving. I found the work gentle but quite demanding and surprisingly strengthening.

Benefits

Although Feldenkrais is not a treatment for specific physical disorders, people with neuromuscular problems, such as strokes, multiple sclerosis and cerebral palsy are sometimes referred to Feldenkrais practitioners for individual lessons. Benefits for everyone generally include:

- improving posture
- improving voice projection, quality and pitch
- easing pain in the back, neck and shoulders
- learning how to avoid repetitive strain injury
- improving self-awareness in presentation skills in the workplace
- developing greater awareness and flexibility.

Contraindications

Feldenkrais doesn't work for people who want to be fixed or cured without work/participation/awareness of their own. It also doesn't work very well if you are extremely speedy and don't enjoy slowing down for a little while.

Dance movement therapy

'Through dance and all the arts we can make profound connections with ourselves and develop deeper and more satisfying contact and communication with others' (Rosa Shreeves).[14]

Throughout the ages dance has always been a part of healing rituals. It was during the 1940s that dance therapy began to be developed in psychiatry. Marion Chace, a pioneer in this field, was one of the first dance therapists to work successfully with patients at St Elizabeth's Hospital, Washington DC, US. Nowadays Dance Movement Therapy (often known as DMT) is used broadly in the public sector, such as in schools, hospitals, and day-care centres, as well as within private practice with individuals and groups. DMT encompasses a wide range of psychotherapeutic approaches. In this form of bodywork the insights that a person gains comes from the movement itself; it is the movement that is the language.

Through 'reawakening our awareness of how our body feels' and how it moves we can reach greater physical and emotional freedom, a lessening of anxiety and constriction. We can find a new sense of flexibility, strength and a greater responsiveness to others and to our environment. Our intuition can become sharper and we can increase our sense of choice and possibility so that we can 'feel more fully functioning and alive.'[15]

Even ten or fifteen minutes of moving the body – just following how we feel it wants to move – at the beginning of the day makes a huge difference to how much energy we have available. You don't need to be in a class or movement therapy group, you can be with your own natural movement. However, you may choose to join one and this will certainly deepen your experience. As Katya Bloom and Rosa Shreeves say in their book *Moves*, 'Many people are familiar with feeling out of touch with their bodies and therefore out of touch with themselves. All too often we are "thinking heads", carrying our bodies around like suitcases, mostly unaware of them unless they break down.'[16] This book is a wonderful source book of ideas for body awareness and creative movement, and indicates how it moves very easily into dance.

Dance movement therapists use a wide range of dance and improvisation structures to support their client in finding her own movements, expression and self-development. You may choose this form of therapy because you want to explore a physical symptom, such as a stiff neck. Alternatively, you may have a desire for movement, or want to explore a particular issue such as the emotion of jealousy, or how you go about making friends with someone; or you may explore elemental images such as wind or fire. Often in a session a particular theme or topic may be chosen or may arise spontaneously. The movement itself, such as moving high or low, jumping, or crawling and so on, can be the source of spontaneous expression.

In DMT you explore feelings, patterns of behaviour and your relationship to yourself and those around you. The way that the therapist works will be very varied and she will be responsive to each individual and group. There may be particular emphasis on the physical, emotional or spiritual aspects of the work according to the needs of the client and the personal style of the therapist.

DMT is concerned with the expression of the language of the body. Anita Green writes, 'Overall it is a valuable, and at times cathartic, medium for expressing feelings – feelings perhaps too overwhelming to put into words.'[17] All sorts of things are revealed through moving in this way and we can become conscious of patterns of movement and behaviour in our lives. Part of the healing comes from sharing the experience with the therapist and with others if you are in a group. Although the advantages of DMT may be far ranging, as a result of doing it you may well feel much physically fitter and more in charge of your life.

Personal physical and emotional safety is an inherent element within DMT. The therapist will be observing her client or clients very closely and one of her tasks is to take care of those she is working with. People are encouraged to work within their own range of movements and keep themselves safe in the class.

Caroline is a single woman, aged thirty-three years. She began DMT three and a half years ago. She first went for weekly sessions and later reduced it to twice a month. She is now planning to further reduce the number of sessions. She works one to one with her therapist in her therapist's studio:

'Within the therapeutic space created with my dance movement therapist I have started to integrate my thoughts with my bodily feelings and sensations. Alongside this process DMT has allowed me to respect my outer layer, ie my skin, as a place where I begin and end, a place of comfort. In turn I've been able to reassess my own bodily definition. My body has empowered me and helped me to decide who I am, what I want and what I choose not to have for myself. Of course this healing process has been greatly facilitated by the therapeutic space coupled with my therapist, who has used her body in relation to mine. For example, she has used a mirroring technique to help me understand my body. By reflecting back to me using her own body I have seen how I move in historical patterns. In looking at her body, which is my body, I've been able to create different ways of being.

DMT has empowered me to listen to the subtleties of my body, to hear its tension, excitement and history. My history is mapped on to the surface of my body. Its physiological strength has allowed me to safely unravel the complexities of myself.'

Gabrielle Roth five rhythms movement practice

Gabrielle Roth, an American dancer, has spent her life studying dance, theatre and the healing arts. She has developed a form of movement that is both free-style dance and, when entered deeply, can become a source for our own dance art and healing. 'Given our concentration, focus and commitment to the practice, this work can become a life journey which catalyses the whole psyche into motion' (Roland Wilkinson and Susanne Perks of Second Wave, see Resources).

The Five Rhythms provide a structure for the exploration of our own unique dance and constitute a complete range of movement and expression. These are flow, staccato, chaos, lyrical rhythm and stillness. Roth believes that it is essential for health on all levels that we can access and learn to let these rhythms emerge:

- flow is about moving confidently and with ease in the world, being able to trust, take in and use what nourishes us most
- staccato involves percussive movements, creating boundaries, knowing where your body ends and some else's begins. This is the embodiment of being able to communicate honestly and simply
- chaos involves being able to move through the surprises, contradictions and paradoxes of life and experiencing these as challenges rather than threats
- lyrical rhythm can be very moving, supporting you to be moved to tears or laughter or other forms of expression that bring us comfort
- stillness is about not being stuck or inert but vibrant and coming from a place in ourselves of trust and love.

These rhythms are within everyone and each one moves you in physically different ways, encouraging the direct emergence of movement within your body, emotions and thinking. The process initiates freedom in our dance and can change the way we experience ourselves and the world around us. It is not dependent on how much or how little a person is able to move and everyone – young people, grandparents, people in wheelchairs – can free their body a little bit more.

This practice is useful to those who have hardly danced at all as well as to experienced students of movement and dance. Age is no barrier. No one is either too experienced to learn or has the 'wrong' body shape to dance.

Judy Hargreaves, a fifty-two-year-old mother of two, combines drumming and dance. She writes:

I experience Gabrielle Roth's work as very powerful and supportive in doing my own dance. Both this and working and focusing on my process of learning African drumming get me out of my head. Drumming is definitely bodywork for me. When

I was getting over flu recently and it was too cold to go outside for a few days I danced to Five Rhythms for an hour a day which really helped me connect to the ground and move my healing on.'

Self-help
It's good to do regular body awareness movement or dance, every day if you can. You may begin with some gentle rolling of your neck to loosen it and follow this with rotating your shoulders, working with one and then the other. Very soon the rest of your body 'starts to tell you' which parts it wants to move, so you may start rotating your torso from the hips and ease out any tension in your pelvis. Sometimes you might move very slowly, as slowly as you can. Then you may feel the need to do something more vigorous, such as jumping or running on the spot. When I do this I usually use music and choose what I fancy. Try to be mindful of your body the whole time and allow it to express itself. Sometimes you may feel a sound inside of you, so let it come out. Sometimes, if this is an angry sound, it is showing you that you have some frustration in your body that you had no idea was there.

If you have a physical symptom you can 'dance' it: move as if you are that symptom. Or you may dance out a dream, memory or particular mood. This can be extremely freeing and leave you feeling lighter and happier.

Chapter Eleven

Convergence Therapies

Some therapies are so much on the interface of physical structure, metaphysics, and emotional process that they, as yet, defy categorisation. I have called them 'convergence' therapies, although this does not feel an adequate term. We could call them 'bridging' therapies, but again they are much more than bridges in themselves. The whole is always greater than the sum of its parts. All the therapies here involve gentle, sometimes light, touch.

Rosen method®

'If you do not let yourself be the way you are, your body cannot function. The same is true for the emotions. The only way you can be who you are is through surrender and self-acceptance' Marion Rosen.[1]

Marion Rosen was born in Nuremberg, Germany. In the early 1940s she emigrated to Sweden and then to the US, barely escaping the holocaust. She settled in the San Francisco area where she continues her work. The Rosen Institute was formed in America in 1983.

Two of her teachers in Germany had been Lucy and Dr Gustav Heyer. The latter was a colleague and former student of Jung. The Heyers were members of a group of people in

Munich using massage, breath work and relaxation in conjunction with psychoanalysis. Through bringing together these several disciplines, the treatment time for psychoanalysis could often be reduced considerably. Following on from this Rosen pursued formal training in physical therapy and continued her lifelong interest in dance.

Through fifty years of experience as a physiotherapist, Marion Rosen developed a method of touch based upon her realisation that repressed feelings limit the individual's capacity to breathe fully, thus creating chronic tension in the body. This method works with those muscles that are held, to bring about a physical and emotional awareness. With gentle and unobtrusive touch the practitioner awakens an awareness of tension. Repressed feelings are given the chance to surface into consciousness and be acknowledged. This leads to deep relaxation and a sense of contact with the authentic self.

I like the Marion Rosen approach to the 'unconscious or sub-conscious mind.'[2] She refers to this part of our consciousness as that which is outside of conscious awareness, not 'below' it. To me this takes the drama out of 'hidden' and 'sub' conscious.

This method places particular emphasis on the role of the emotions because Rosen found over and over again in her work that through relaxation it is the emotions that emerge. 'Because mind and body are inextricably linked, Rosen practitioners reach for each through the other. Their particular talent is affecting the mind and body by contact with the body. The point of entry to the system is through the body.'[3]

An important part of the philosophy is that the practitioner does not *do* anything to the client, but serves instead as a facilitator to self-awareness and the subsequent changes that take place in one's life. 'Through contact with the tight muscles, often called barriers, the practitioner meets the holding at its own level, as though reminding the muscle that it is holding and that it has the inherent possibility of relaxing.

The client's awareness follows the practitioner's hands, and relaxation becomes an option.'[4]

I am reminded of the intelligence of the body-mind described in Chapter 1 and life's continuous pulsation of contracting and letting go. These concepts are found in other therapies of different kinds, such as Keleman's Formative Psychology, TRAGER® and TAI CHI.

Reaction during treatment varies widely. For some it is a pleasant, meditative experience, while others will laugh, cry or talk. The body will allow only that which is ready to be expressed.

Benefits

This method is particularly good if:

- you suffer from tense and aching muscles
- you experience difficulty in relaxing
- you feel tired without knowing why
- you want to reach a deeper body awareness
- you want an increased self-knowledge

Here is Brenda's story:

'In my personal process, my experience of the Rosen Method® was of a powerful and benevolent tool. It was akin to being heard at a sensitive and effective level, a way of contacting within my own body what only my body could tell me.

It was direct but not confrontational. It felt like a partnership, the practitioner always asking for permission to touch me and explaining what she saw or noticed as she worked. I felt that no intrusion was possible with such respect shown for my autonomous choices each step of the way. The sensitivity of the practitioner seemed to lead her to locate and identify parts of my body where my life flow was restricted or congested and to speak to the pain in some way through her touch. My body would answer and there would often be an immediate sense of relief.

It was as if in the course of the sessions my body yielded up the terrible sorrow, fear, anger and longing I had felt as a child, with no intellectualisation and sometimes expressed in raw, childish words. This would not have been possible for me if, from the very first touch, the practitioner had not somehow communicated to my body a sense of safety and immense respect. I felt part of a universe that was concrete and clean, as if the right to be in my body had been firmly restored. It felt light, safe, free and at peace and there was often a strong sense of the divine.'

Zero balancing

Zero Balancing (ZB) is hands-on bodywork practised with the recipient clothed and lying on her back on a treatment couch. The mode of touch used enables physical structure and body energy to be engaged simultaneously in a way that harmonises the relationship between them. 'The working focus in Zero Balancing is the interface between the structure of the bones, joints and soft tissues and the energy flowing through them.'[5] This is a significant bridging between the mechanical structural approaches to bodywork and the recognition of vital energy. Hence the difficulty in categorising ZB. What also differentiates ZB from other hands-on therapies is its focus on the most fundamental level of our structure: the bones. On a spiritual level as a recipient you can feel the very essence of your being contacted through your bones.

Zero Balancing was developed from around 1973 by Dr Fritz Smith, an American physician, ACUPUNCTURIST and OSTEOPATH. Fritz Smith believes that by touching in a particular way the energy and the structure of the body can be contacted together. Zero Balancing can bring clearer, stronger force fields of energy into the person. Practitioners have to have recognised qualifications in other forms of healthcare such as ACUPUNCTURE, OSTEOPATHY, CHIROPRACTIC and PHYSIOTHERAPY, before they train.

ZB focuses on particular joints, called foundation joints, where imbalances may occur. A constant process of evaluating, balancing and re-evaluating the structure (joints and ligaments) and energy of the body is made. Using finger pressure and held stretches, the ZB practitioner invites a point of stillness — called a fulcrum — around which the body can relax, creating the opportunity for you to let go of unease and pain and experience a new level of integration.

The actual name, Zero Balancing, came from a client's description of her experience: 'I feel so perfectly balanced; it's almost like I am zero balanced.' A client usually has three sessions at weekly intervals to allow the work to consolidate and build. If you want to deepen the experience you could continue sessions at perhaps three or four weekly intervals. You might also choose to go from time to time as you felt the need.

Modes of contact that the Zero Balancer uses are defined as follows:

- Blending: the deliberate blurring of the boundary between your energetic body and another's. There is a fusion between yours and another's field. This approach is used in SUBTLE ENERGY HEALING and CRANIO-SACRAL THERAPY.
- Streaming: where the practitioner directs her own energy to flow into her client. She may be intending to direct energy along a meridian to an acupuncture point or to a particular chakra. In this situation the energy comes directly from the practitioner's energy. This can happen in SUBTLE ENERGY HEALING.

- Channelling: the practitioner opens herself to forces beyond herself so that she becomes a conduit for others. Again, this happens in SUBTLE ENERGY HEALING.
- Interface: the practitioner maintains clear energetic and structural boundaries where she ends and her client begins.

Benefits

ZB is excellent for sports people, those who don't like deep manipulation and those who like to keep their clothes on. It is particularly successful for headaches, neck and shoulder pain and lower back problems. It can bring increased flexibility in the body, and can help our ability to adapt to life's stresses and changes. Is very good for people wanting to increase their sense of well-being.

Contraindications

ZB is not for those with knee replacements, epilepsy, MS or cancer, recent fractures, recovering from recent major surgery or illness; people with schizophrenia or other mental disturbance.

Jenny Stanton is in her late forties, a divorced mother of two:

'I'd never heard of Zero Balancing before and so I booked for my first session in a spirit of curiosity. One of the things that appealed to me was the idea that it was something you could have even if you were well, like massage; a kind of treat. I didn't think I needed any "therapy" (even though in fact I was pretty stressed by work and unsorted about relationships). Also I liked the idea of "balancing", of paying attention to my body and integrating it with my mind. For ages, my body had been like a workhorse that had to be fed and stabled but whose job was just to haul me around. My head was the only part that had seemed important.

The pattern of the initial session was the same as for all the subsequent ones. First Pam (my ZB therapist) talked to me, asking how I was and recording points in a notebook. (She quite often comes back to these in a later session and asks how I've got on with, say, my headaches or some other slight problem that I may have forgotten because I've followed her advice and overcome it. Or not.) Next, she got me to sit on the edge of the couch and rock to either side while she felt the place where the spine joins the pelvis. Then I lay down on my back – with my clothes on – and she literally pulled my legs. Not suddenly; with a steady traction so I felt a bit longer.

She felt all down my spine, each side of the bony protuberances, and then pressed quite hard, upwards into the sacrum. I had an extraordinary, strong sensation as if a stream of fluid was running down from that point inside my back bone, while the place she pressed was flying up higher than a hilltop. (This never happened again so strongly.) She gently manipulated my legs, concentrating on the hip and knee joints, and then worked on my feet. She spent less time on my arms, but she gave my shoulder blades and neck a good deal of attention.

It was quite different from a massage because the focus was on the joints. Besides various tingling sensations, which I enjoyed, it produced a profound feeling of peace, of letting go. I booked in for another session. I didn't know what it was doing but it felt good.

Above all, in that first session, I experienced a series of – I don't know what to call them – visions. Images of places I had been, but so vivid that it seemed I was actually there, each one produced by Pam's movement or pressure on a different part of my body. I remember one: she pressed on my breastbone and, while I felt her touch at one level, at another I was standing in the misty rain at Chysausester, an ancient British settlement in Cornwall. I could see the stones overgrown with moss, smell the wet ferns. It was as though I were in a trance almost from the beginning of the 'hands-on' part of the session. Afterwards I said to Pam that I'd been in all sorts of places but she didn't comment much, so I didn't know if this was common or my particular response to ZB. I think she said people respond in lots of different ways. She also warned me not to do too much after the session, even if I felt a burst of energy; some people do, although others feel tired.

As I had more sessions and learned a bit more about ZB, I realised it's a lot to do with energy: Pam would mention different types of energy, or conjure up an image of energy blocked like a river facing a dam. So I came to see that my unsatisfactory life was hampering the free flow of my energies. Yet I continued with things as they were, by and large, apart from going to ZB, which seemed to do me good. I'd talk about making some major changes and Pam would encourage me, but I didn't do it. I was frightened to do anything too drastic. My head was still in charge.

Then my back went. It was associated with the strain of commuting from Oxford to London for work about three times a week. It got better, it got worse. There was a terrible period of six or seven months of chronic pain, often quite disabling, though not severe enough to stop me going to work. In the midst of this, after a particularly bad (painful in several senses) week away with the man who I'd been seeing on and off for four years, I had an amazing ZB session. (I somehow knew I had to go despite the pain that made it hard to lie on my back.) As usual I relaxed into a sort of trance when Pam worked on my spine. Then the place-hallucinations started: I was struggling up to the top of Masatiompan, a mountain in the west of Ireland, in a terrible thick fog and driving rain. This continued for a while; I started down the other side, slipping in the mud on the steep hillside, falling on my bum. Pam moved on and I was transported to different, more ordinary places. Towards the end, as she was moving my head, I felt I was on top of another mountain, in the Alps, coming round a corner with a glorious view of Mount Rosa and the Matterhorn. The air was pure and the snowy mountain peaks sparkled in the clear light. I came out of that session determined not to mess around with/be messed around by that man any longer.

Perhaps the only vision that wasn't of some place I'd been was of tidewater swirling in a dock; trapped, angry water, rather like the lock water in a canal when they open the upper gates.

The more intractable problem in my life was around my work, and the commuting. My back pain seemed caught up with that. I don't expect ZB or any "therapy" to resolve my dilemmas for me but, as with the stuck relationship, I think in the long run ZB may help me to move on. It helps me to be in touch with intuitive parts of myself; something I have found very difficult if not impossible for most of my life. It works quite obliquely for me, associated with these place-images that don't directly tell me anything but seem somehow nourishing. I come out of a session feeling incredibly calm and restored, always an immediate benefit.

Pam herself is a wonderful advertisement for her techniques. About my age, she looks younger because she's both peaceful and vital. She goes on courses to learn more about ZB and is involved in training other people in the method; there's quite an international network. With her wise advice on all sorts of issues, and her communicative hands, she has helped me to start integrating my strangely split life.'

The Bowen technique: Bowtech®

This technique was pioneered by Tom Bowen of Geelong, Victoria, Australia. Tom Bowen died in 1982 and his work was carried on by an osteopath, Oswald Rentsch, and his wife

Elaine. Apparently Tom Bowen alone treated thirteen thousand patients a year, ninety per cent of whom only required two or three treatments – exceptional claims indeed! Elaine and Oswald Rentsch were commissioned by Tom Bowen to document his work and they have introduced the technique into many countries, with the UK being the most recent.

The Bowen Technique has been described as 'physical homoeopathy' (see Appendix II). It involves a series of light moves across muscles, tendons and ligaments throughout the body. This work on the superficial fascia results in the same significant changes deep and often painful stroking provides. Light, but firm pressure is used, using thumb and fingers to roll the muscle and create a vibrational disturbance within the body. There is no manipulation or adjustment of hard tissue and the treatment is very gentle, subtle and relaxing. The technique allows the body to do the work required to heal itself without imposing the will of the therapist on to the patient. The therapist treats the patient not the condition.

The treatment can be done through light clothing and is very gentle. It is therefore very good for children, older and disabled people. During a session the therapist leaves the room for short periods in order to allow the information coming through the touch to be assimilated into the body. Many clients report a deep state of relaxation and a sense of 'things moving' when left alone.

There are a number of possible theories as to how the method works. It can be said that sickness, injury or disease is just a lack of communication between brain and body. If this balance is restored then anything is possible. The gentle moves made by the therapist prompt the body to examine its systems via receptors and nerve endings and simply exchange information with the brain. Once the brain knows there is a problem it will sort it out. It is a form of cellular communication; each cell is a miniature wireless tuned in to the frequency of the body. When certain parts are out of tune then illness or injury result. Retuning means that the body heals itself. Similar to SPIRITUAL or SUBTLE ENERGY HEALING, the therapist is a conduit (see Chapter 8).

The therapy is offered to the body and the body then decides how best to use it. Bowtech is not a replacement for medical advice, but a chance for the patient's body to make a choice, rather than having a set of sometimes arbitrary interventions thrust upon it.

Benefits
Bowtech is used by midwives during labour. It can be used for newborn babies, and the elderly. It is good for:

- back pain
- frozen shoulder
- tennis elbow
- asthma
- whiplash injury
- sports injuries
- hayfever and bronchial symptoms
- carpal tunnel syndrome (compression of the main nerve supply to the hand)
- RSI (repetitive strain injury)
- general relaxation and body balancing.

Contraindications
There is one move that is not used during pregnancy.

Suze Morton, aged fifty-three, is a mother of two grown-up children and has been a nurse since she was seventeen years old.

'Approximately sixteen years ago I was diagnosed by a neurologist as having carpal tunnel syndrome in both hands.

This is basically a compression of the main nerve supply to the hand, which decreases the nerves' blood supply and causes sensations like pins and needles in the hands and forearms, intermittent pain in the fingers and thumbs and muscle wastage in the hands. Eventually, once my children had grown, I decided to try an orthodox treatment; a surgical operation on my right hand. Some three months later the condition had not improved so I cancelled the planned operation for the left hand and decided to try alternative therapies.

I visited a chiropractor who decided to try the Bowen technique. This was an entirely pleasant experience, not at all painful and very gentle. It involved moving the skin across a muscle and then, with a light pressure, pulling it back across the muscle. Somehow, this seemed to release something and over a period of four weekly treatments the condition greatly improved.

If I get any symptoms now I have another treatment and this usually sorts out the problem. I believe if I had had this treatment many years earlier the condition would be entirely cured. Having had the symptoms for many years and not doing anything about it a certain amount of permanent damage has been done to the nerves.'

Trager® approach

This approach, also known as Psychophysical Integration and Mentastics® Movement Education, was the discovery of Milton Trager. He was born in 1908 in the US. In the 1930s, when he was a young boxer and acrobat living in Miami, Florida, he decided that rather than keep pushing himself to his physical limits, he would see what it would be like to jump and then land in the softest possible way. In doing this, he changed his whole thinking from aiming for maximum effort to seeking maximum effortlessness, and this became his life's work. He developed a series of sensitive, gentle movements, such as rocking and stretching, to bring about a feeling of ease and comfort to others. He later trained as a medical doctor in order to give his form of bodywork a scientific basis.

The words used for this approach are interesting. Stretching and rocking are fairly straightforward to imagine, but practitioners also do what is called rolling, bouncing and shimmering. Rolling is a backwards and forwards movement, rather like how you would use a rolling pin or how a cradle moves. Bouncing is a 'sending out and returning' movement like the bouncing of a ball. This is also to do with compression; for example, if you push down on to a balloon it changes shape and when you let go it bounces back. Rolling and bouncing are used on a limb; for example, your leg will be held and gently bounced. Shimmering is very soothing for the central nervous system. It involves the practitioner moving her hand very swiftly, but extremely softly, backwards and forwards over a muscle or group of muscles. In this approach nothing is forced, nothing hurts.

Agni Eckroyd, a UK Trager practitioner, describes this re-education process: 'Rather than trying to go in and fix problems, we try to show the body how it could be more comfortable, more flexible, more easy... It's like talking to the mind within the body. The practitioner never asserts her idea of how soft or free an area should be; she deliberately retreats from such assertions and instead projects through the motions of her hands the questions, "What can be lighter and freer than that? Yes. And lighter than that? Fine. And freer than that?" And so on.'

A Trager session usually lasts one and a half hours, during which the client receives several thousand light, rhythmical touches. 'You leave the couch feeling as if you have been rocked like a child secure in its mother's arms.'[6] As the client you choose how often you go for a session, maybe fortnightly or every few months. You need time to integrate the experience.

In March 1998 I received just a fifteen-minute 'taster' Trager session at a complementary therapies exhibition and loved it. The idea is that the body is re-educated into remembering the experience of pleasure rather than pain. Rather like the metaphysical healing methods, the Trager practitioner works in a relaxed meditative state of consciousness. Dr Trager calls this 'hook-up'. This way of being means that the practitioner can connect very deeply with the recipient in an unforced way, remaining continually aware of the slightest responses. It also means the practitioner can work effectively without getting tired herself.

The physiological effects are that, with relaxation, pain can be eased for numerous conditions. Apart from the relaxation effects it also promotes greater flexibility of the joints. Because the gentle rocking movements radiate through the whole body the internal organs also receive attention, making it an extremely deep feeling experience.

The Mentastics® part of the session is the learning you do to help yourself. These are movements that help to recreate the sensations you experienced during the session. They are referred to as 'mental gymnastics'. For example, as I sit here typing I can catch myself feeling tense, stop for a second and ask myself 'How long is my spine?' In simply asking this question – without needing a particular answer and with no judgments such as 'I ought to sit up straighter' – I am automatically rising out of my slumped posture. I can then ask, 'How loving can I be to my spine?' (My actual answer right now is to take a break, which I have been putting off for half an hour!)

Deane Juhan, Trager instructor, says, 'It is a means of teaching the client to recall the pleasurable sensory state which produced positive tissue change, and because it is this feeling state which triggered positive tissue response in the first place, every time the feeling is clearly recalled the changes can deepen, become more permanent, and the client becomes more receptive to further positive change.'[7] This is a relatively new therapy in the UK but one that I think will grow. At the moment practitioners are largely around the south coast, but with annual UK-based trainings, Trager membership is now growing nationally. Trainings are also available in other countries.

Describing the Trager® approach I am reminded a little of the ALEXANDER TECHNIQUE in that this is not a medical treatment, it is a learning experience. The recipient is learning what it is like to be freer and lighter in the body and to feel integrated, coordinated and connected to the energies that sustain you. Mentastics can be adapted to help in any activity in your daily life.

Contraindications
The Trager® approach would not be used where there is active thrombosis phlebitis, recent surgery (up to three months), the early stages of pregnancy, inflamed arthritis and certain cancers. Where there is a serious or chronic medical condition practitioners should always seek the permission of a person's doctor before giving sessions.

Self-help
Mentastics® or 'mental gymnastics' involve using the mind and developing bodily awareness. In addition to my own example above, here is an example taken from an article by health journalist Jane Alexander:

Think about softening and widening; think about expanding and lengthening your body. Think about being lighter. You can let one arm drop down at your side and let your fingers waggle. Notice the weight of the arm. As you relax it be aware of what happens, it may actually lengthen. Do the same on the other side.

While seated imagine that your head is attached to the ceiling by a large rubber band. Notice how that affects you; your posture may become straighter, but not stiff. Feel your shoulders soften and drop down as your head bobs on the elastic. Now imagine that you have a paintbrush fixed to the top of your head and that you are gently painting the ceiling with it. With tiny movements let your head wobble from side to side.

The metamorphic technique

'Life is creation and from creation comes movement: that movement is change, and it is the life force that sustains this change within the many differing cycles of existence, be it a tree, a planet or a human being... The metamorphic technique stresses that even beyond this life force, the principle with which practitioners work is, simply, life.'[8]

Historically this technique has its roots in REFLEXOLOGY and zone therapy. However, in the 1960s, a naturopath called Robert St John came to realise that the stresses that lead to illness fall into two distinct categories: those that pull away from life and those that push too forcefully into life. Having studied reflexology he developed his own treatment, being drawn particularly to observing the psychological effects. This technique is a fascinating form of light-touch massage, the focus of which primarily is the feet. Practitioners also work on the hands and the head.

What is different about the metamorphic technique is that it is concerned with life before we are born. It is believed that the growth of the embryo corresponds to the development of consciousness. The embryo develops from the brain down to the base of the spine, and then from the spine outwards to the limbs. It is during the nine months of gestation that the potentials of human life are established.

It has been found that by working on the spinal reflexes of the feet, hands and head, this formative period, including the influences of preconception, conception, post-conception, quickening, pre-birth and birth, is brought back into focus and something called the 'time structure' is loosened. This time structure refers to the points in time at which aspects of the embryo's development are 'held'. Since life itself is not bound by time, space or matter then the work can be done 'out of time'. This involves the practitioner 'getting themselves out of the way'; that is, not imposing any kind of direction on the work. It is the life force of the receiver that knows what to do to become well or more whole or to reach greater potential. The work itself is not goal oriented. In this way the metamorphic technique is similar to HEALING (see Chapter 8).

It is believed that through this work it is the essential life force of the receiver that releases the energies that were impeded during the prenatal period. We are, in essence, the consciousness that is developed during gestation, as a result of all the influences present at the time of our conception. These influences may be parental, cultural, or environmental. They may be to do with the evolutionary stage that humans have reached, and be to do with more cosmic influences.

Because the work focuses on this early time in our development it is used especially for children and adults with learning difficulties and for those with physical disabilities.

The metamorphic technique practitioner is not primarily concerned with symptoms and this makes it different from many other therapies. Rather, the individual is viewed as perfect just as she is and at the same time she has a life force that is working towards fulfilling her potential as a human being. No one can ever know what that is for another person.

The technique is easy to learn and can be given by anyone to any other person. It is taught to people with learning disabilities so that they can give it to others. It involves massaging lightly, with the balls of the fingers, along the side of the instep of the foot and over the top of the foot from ankle to ankle. On the hands the pattern follows from the top of the thumb down to the wrist and over the wrist. On the head it involves massaging from the centre of the brow over the top of the head and along each side of the base of the skull.

When you receive this technique you usually lie down, or sit at right angles to the practitioner, and have your feet bare. You place one foot in your practitioner's lap. You may even be watching television or reading. You may want to talk or relax; it makes no difference. Although the process is simple, and you may think nothing much is happening, the effect can be quite profound. I feel there is an abstract nature to this therapy that can make it is difficult for the intellect to grasp. After receiving this kind of massage I have felt deeply connected with myself as if I have a 'right' place in the universe.

Pulsing

Pulsing can be described as a 'massage in motion', and has its roots in TRAGER® work and Huna Bodywork (see Appendix II). It is a deeply enjoyable form of bodywork combining movements of stretching, lifting and rotating with a continuous rhythmic rocking. It has been available in London at least since the early 1980s.

Guy Gladstone and Silke Ziehl, two long-standing therapists at the Open Centre in London, are practitioners and trainers in this therapy. They were both taught in 1978 by

Curtis Turchin, a postural integration trainer and Trager practitioner from California. Curtis has coined the term 'Pulsing' to present his extension of traditional Trager technique. Pulsing relocates Tragering in the context of the neo-Reichian therapies (see Chapter 9).

In his article 'Pulsing – Massage in Motion' Guy Gladstone describes the field of pulses within which we live: 'The heartbeat itself; the pulse of the bloodstream, held by the muscular walls of the veins and arteries; the elastic and layered qualities of those channels... the circulation of lymph; the finer pulses of meridian energy familiar to acupuncturists; and the pulsating quality of breathing... Consider too a meaning of impulse, a movement of energy from the core of a body towards its surface. In a body free to feel, impulses translate into emotions.'[9]

The practitioner of pulsing begins by imparting a rhythmic movement with one or both hands. Often one hand is used as the 'mother' hand, gently holding and supporting, and the other as the moving hand. The practitioner begins to make a relationship with the whole field of pulses latent within you as she gently moves you from side to side with rocking and rolling movements. A steady rhythm builds up, and you allow yourself to be moved from both without and within.

My own experience of receiving a pulsing session many years ago remains a strong, pleasant memory. I felt gently rocked, each part of my body receiving exactly the right amount of contact and stimulation. I relaxed very deeply and felt as if I was floating in a womb-like space. It was very good indeed!

Ashley Montague describes the use of the cradle in the history of child rearing, and how important rocking is in providing tactile stimulation. He suggests that people who rock themselves are replicating the natural rocking of the foetus in the womb. Rocking has a self-comforting value, and in certain cultures is common during prayer or mourning. 'Rocking in both babies and adults increases cardiac output and is helpful to the circulation; it promotes respiration and discourages lung congestion. It stimulates muscle tone and, also importantly, it maintains the feeling of relatedness. A baby, especially, that is rocked, knows that it is not alone. A general cellular and visceral stimulation results from the rocking.'[10]

When emotional issues surface pulsing lends itself to being combined with other therapies, such as BIO-ENERGETICS, GESTALT, and CREATIVE VISUALISATION.

Conclusion

My own experience of a number of bodywork therapies (including body psychotherapy, neo-Reichian and Gestalt, rebirthing, massage, healing, cranial osteopathy and yoga) described in this book has been so life changing it is difficult to put into words. I also use other CAM therapies, especially homoeopathy, nutritional therapy and magnetic therapy (see Appendix II). I want to include these because I owe my present wellness to them, too, not just bodywork therapies. I believe I would not have been able to reach my present level of physical wellness, emotional stability and spiritual fulfilment without them. My own healing process over the last twenty or more years has been and continues to be a journey of discovery.

Overall, the women who have contributed to this book have been very positive about the therapies they have tried and they have been helped considerably. Sometimes a therapy seems not to to have helped at all and some people with chronic, serious, painful conditions have tried a host of therapies and have found varying degrees of help. But for thousands of women these therapies have changed their lives fundamentally for the better. What is clear is that often our beliefs and our relationship to our own health, the therapy and the therapist are integral to benefits we gain.

Sarah writes:

'I have been greatly helped by the different therapies I have tried. I would be very careful about seeking therapy from someone without a personal recommendation. It seems to me a great pity that these therapies are not available unless you can pay for them. My GP was very welcoming of the idea of me going for acupuncture and I would like to think that more doctors might see the complementarity of complementary medicine. All of the people I have consulted have been very professional, have belonged to a professional association and have kept records in a way that affirms my confidence in them.'

To have access to a wide variety of therapies broadens the possibilities of relief from suffering immensely. My hope is that this book will inspire you to seek and find what is right for you. I wish you the best possible life you can have.

Appendix I

The following is a detailed comparison between conventional medicine and CAM. The aim is to provide some understanding of the shift that I believe needs to take place in the theoretical models, philosophy, consciousness and behaviour within the professional relationship between doctor and patient. Although changes are taking place there is still a chasm between these two kinds of approach, and the public misses out on receiving help and information that exists outside the medical institutions.

These points are polarised to some extent to highlight the contrast. The medical profession is becoming increasingly influenced by the holistic approach. On the other hand some CAM practitioners can still be very influenced by their own conditioning in the medical model and behave as if they know better than their patient or client.

Philosophy

In conventional medicine the approach is specialised, with the physical body being divided into many parts. The focus of knowledge and research has become more and more refined and this continues to be the case. In CAM the concern is with the whole person. Each aspect of the physical body is integrated as much as possible, as is the emotional, mental and spiritual life of the patient or client. The emphasis is on achieving maximum wellness.

Belief

Within conventional medicine, and within science generally, the belief is that everything is explainable. Within CAM, although understanding is sought, mystery is allowable and is seen as part of the human experience.

Emphasis

In conventional medicine the emphasis is on efficiency. This leads to an institutionalised system and control of the individual. In part this is due to the sheer numbers of patients requiring attention. Within CAM the emphasis is on human values and what it feels like to be the recipient of the treatment. This is helped by the fact that CAM is still largely not available within the primary health care system but is confined to the private sector, so that practitioners see fewer patients or clients in a day and spend much more time with them in sessions.

How the physical body is viewed

In conventional medicine the body is viewed as a machine in good or bad repair, whereas within CAM the body is seen as a dynamic system that exists within a social and cultural context. It is made up of dynamic energy fields and is an organic, intelligent and self-repairing totality.

How the disease or disability is viewed

In conventional medicine disease or disability is seen as a thing, or an entity. In CAM it is seen as a process, through which purpose and meaning may come to light or be discovered.

Focus of treatment or help given

In conventional medicine the main focus is on the treatment of symptoms, which are viewed as wholly negative and to be eradicated at all costs. The primary interventions are allopathic drugs or surgery or both. In CAM, patterns of totalities are looked for. Symptoms are viewed as information about conflict or disharmony. They are seen as the body's response to external or internal distress and are often a reflection of the body attempting to heal itself. Technology is minimal and techniques used are non-invasive as possible.

Use of data

In conventional medicine the primary reliance is on quantitative information, such as charts, tests and dates, with an increasing reliance on technology. The emphasis is on acquiring a body of clinical information that is right and can be relied on. Within CAM the primary reliance is on qualitative information, including the patient or client's subjective reports and the professional's intuition. Quantitative data is a valuable adjunct. The emphasis is on learning how to listen to the patient, and being open to and evaluating new concepts.

The role of the mind

In conventional medicine the body and mind are separate with the mind being a secondary factor in organic illness. In CAM the mind is viewed as primary or co-equal in the causation and recovery from illness, and psychosomatic symptoms are valued.

Placebo

The placebo effect in conventional medicine demonstrates the power of suggestion, but within CAM it shows how integral the mind's role is to disease and healing.

Health-care worker and the patient/client relationship

In conventional medicine the professional is given a considerable amount of power while the patient is completely dependent on the medical staff. The relationship is generally one of patronage, with the doctor being the ultimate diagnoser and authority. Within CAM the professional should be a therapeutic partner who supports, facilitates and encourages the self-healing and autonomy of the patient or client.

The needs of the health-care worker

In conventional medicine the health-care worker is a detached expert who should be emotionally neutral and outside what is taking place with the patient. She or he is often overworked with little time to spend with patients. The need to process or off-load the emotional responses she or he may have to working with pain and suffering is not encouraged. Within CAM the health-care worker is part of what is taking place and knows that her or his presence is a component of the healing and therefore a major influence on the treatment. The health-care worker's own needs as a professional are acknowledged.

Presence of the professional

Within conventional medicine the medical professional must be present, but with some types of CAM, such as healing and radionics, the patient or client can be helped from a distance.

Prevention

Within conventional medicine prevention tends to be largely environmental, although diet, exercise, and abstinence from smoking are now increasingly emphasised. Within CAM prevention is synonymous with wholeness, and may include rest, exercise, abstinence from smoking, and examination of work patterns, relationships and personal goals. It is much more likely to include the use of vitamins and supplements and in fact nutrition in general. Practices that are seen as essential and safe within conventional medicine and dentistry can be seriously debated within CAM. Examples include the long- and short-term dangers of immunisation, and the detrimental effects of mercury poisoning from amalgam dental fillings. In addition, local and world environmental issues are viewed as part of health care within CAM.

Death

Within conventional medicine death is viewed as failure. Within CAM it is viewed as part of the life process. When death is inevitable, patients or clients can be supported through this transition.

Appendix II

Glossary of bodywork therapies not widely available yet in the UK, plus important alternative and complementary medicine therapies that you may know or have heard of.

Anthroposophical medicine
This is based on the work of Rudolf Steiner, an Austrian scientist and philosopher who believed in reincarnation. Practitioners are medically qualified, but they also view the human being as having four distinct aspects – the physical, the ego or self, and subtle bodies known as the etheric and astral.

Art therapy
A method of self-exploration using art materials. It is very good for finding expression where words are not easy or possible to find.

Ayurvedic medicine
A form of healing from India, used for thousands of years, which combines herbal remedies, massage and diet therapy together with medicine and meditation. It is a way of life. In India it is the main form of medicine, and orthodox doctors, Ayurvedic physicians and homoeopaths work alongside each other.

Bates method
A holistic approach using exercises and techniques for improving eyesight, perception and taking care of the eyes.

Biodanza

Biodanza is a form of dance therapy. 'Bios' means life, and 'danza' means integrated movements full of meaning. Biodanza consequently means 'the dance of life'. Through movement exercises and therapeutic processes it supports people to find new ways of communicating and expressing themselves. The system was created and developed in the 1960s by Rolando Toro Araneda, a lecturer in Psychology and Medical Anthropology at the Catholic University of Santiago, Chile. In 1991 Patricia Martello, helped by Caroline Churba, an English physiotherapist, introduced Biodanza to the UK.

Biofeedback

The use of sensitive electronic instruments to monitor autonomic (ie involuntary) physiological processes. People are trained to tune in to their bodily functions and responses and eventually to learn how to control them.

Biomagnetic therapy

A method that employs the use of small magnets placed on meridians to rebalance energy flow.

Biosynthesis

A form of body psychotherapy, pioneered by a psychotherapist called David Boadella, that is a development of Reich's vegetotherapy. It is influenced by bio-energetics, biodynamic psychotherapy, the Laban method of dance therapy, Stanley Keleman's somatic emotional therapy, the work of psychologist Frank Lake, and the work of subtle anatomy healer Robert Moore.

Body harmony

Body harmony is non-invasive and is often referred to as 'the listening touch'. Like many bodywork therapies it is based on the concept that the memories that shape our being and the way in which we relate, function and create our lives are stored in the tissues of our body. As a therapy it is powerful and pleasurable, and recognises the client as the expert on herself. The practitioner listens with every sense available to her, often using her hands on the body and following the body's wishes or instructions. It can help with the permanent release of many conditions, such as arthritis, addiction and depression. It is also said to be excellent during pregnancy, labour and postnatally.

Buteko Method
Professor KP Buteko, a Russian scientist, discovered in the early twentieth century that dysfunctional breathing can often result in some manifestation of disease. His method involves the retraining of breathing patterns to increase oxygenation of blood and tissues. Research in 1994 in Australia has shown that this method may help asthma sufferers considerably.

Core energetics
Founded by John Pierrakos, a student of Reich, together with his wife Eva Pierrakos, core energetics works to move through and transform the individual's defence system in order to reach the core, a level of consciousness that represents the higher qualities of life, with love being the central expression. This core is called the 'seat of love'. It involves deep work with the body and expanding the consciousness so that the client can discover her main task in this life and so fulfil her destiny. It incorporates many evolutionary healing influences, including basic Reichian concepts, bio-energetics and insights from modern physics. Core energetics maintains that a person is a psychosomatic unity, that the source of healing and capacity to love is within the self and is not outside, and that all existence forms a unity that moves towards a creative evolution. In the human being this evolution consists of deep transformation of the negative aspects of the personality to form a creative whole.

Dream therapy
Practically all forms of psychotherapy offer ways of working with the material of dreams. The dream is viewed as being symbolic. There are several ways of working with dreams. The classical psychoanalytical approach views them retrospectively; that is, the dream material represents what is coming up from the unconscious mind, albeit in a

censored and distorted way. A second way is to see them as being about the present. For instance, a gestalt therapist may work with a dream by inviting her client to become each main item or person in the dream in turn, and to let each one speak to the others and say what it wants. This helps the client grasp how the dream symbolises the relationship between different parts of her psyche. Another way is to view dreams as being about the future. This is a Jungian approach where the dream is viewed as being about our journey towards becoming fully ourselves. It is about our aspirations and directions in life. In Dance Movement Therapy just a particular quality, mood, action or recurring image of a dream can be worked with. As with other approaches, although perhaps more directly, movement can bring you into the feeling sense of dreaming, and you can gain access to flashes of dreams that are locked away.

Describing your dreams literally by writing them down or sharing them with a friend can bring you powerful insights into your own inner personal process. Often problems can be solved through paying attention to our dreams. To 'catch' a dream immediately you wake it is good to have a pen and paper by your bed, or a tape recorder.

Energetic integration

This is an innovative development of REICHIAN WORK by Jack Painter and Wilhelm Poppeliers, rooted in Reich's pioneering work as well as modern therapeutic methods such as bio-energetic analysis, core energetics, gestalt process work and trauma healing. It uses a wide range of mind and body-oriented approaches, including body-sensing, breath work and cycles of charge and discharge, expressive movement, gestalt enactment, body-mind typologies and character analytic processes. It offers a double focus on the individual and on the interpersonal energetic process.

Flotation therapy

This is a method of isolating the body and mind from external stimuli through entering an enclosed tank. The tank contains water, to which have been added minerals and salts to make sure you float easily. The water is kept at skin temperature. The experience brings about deep relaxation, and it has been suggested that one hour of flotation therapy is the equivalent of six hours of sleep.

Flower essences

There are a number of flower essence systems, the most well known being Bach flower therapy and Australian bush flower essences. Remedies are made from the flowers of wild plants, bushes and trees. They work on a vibrational level. For example, each flower essence embodies the harmonious vibrational pattern of the particular flower used, which then resonates and attunes specific energy patterns within human beings. The essences stimulate an enhanced awareness and ability to transform limiting attitudes, emotions and behaviour into more creative, positive and health–affirming ways of living.

G-jo acupressure

A simplified form of ACUPRESSURE, used for immediate relief from many common ailments. In native Chinese it translates as 'first aid'. In ancient China it was used on the battlefields to treat wounded soldiers. Treatment involves a deep, stimulating massage on specific points, working on both sides of the body with the same points. There are 116 small g-jo acupressure points, although the main emphasis is on six close to the feet and hands.

Healing Tao

A sophisticated system of personal energy management based on ancient Chinese philosophy. Techniques include a variety of Taoist meditation and energy practices that increase the flow of chi through the body, drawing in chi from nature, and cleansing and improving the quality of chi in the physical organs.

Hellerwork

Joseph Heller was the former president of the Rolf Institute. He was an aerospace engineer and as such had experience and understanding of structural stress. He studied BIO-ENERGETICS and GESTALT, together with working with other pioneering therapists. He became a ROLFER in 1972 and founded Hellerwork in 1978.

Hellerwork makes the connection between life issues and natural bodily alignment, and shows how to restore the body's natural balance from the inside out. The body is viewed as a hologram of the being. For example, if you cut off the ear from a hologram of an entire face and place the image of the ear in a laser beam, you will not end up with a picture of an ear, but with a picture of a little ear-sized face. Just as the piece of a hologram reflects the entire holographic image, so any part of the body reflects the condition of the entire being: physical, mental, emotional and spiritual. In this way a person's psyche and history can be read by studying the body.

Holotrophic Breathwork®

Holotrophic Breathwork® was developed in 1976 by Stanislav and Christina Grof, leaders in Transpersonal Psychology. In Greek 'holos' means 'whole' or 'complete' and 'trepein' means 'to move in the direction of'. So the term translates as 'moving towards wholeness'. It is a powerful approach involving mobilising the spontaneous healing potential of the body and psyche in unordinary states of consciousness. These states are brought about through techniques of breathing and the use of music and energy-release bodywork. The work can be done individually or in groups. During the sessions all levels of human experience may be accessed, including unfinished issues from postnatal biography and transpersonal phenomena such as psychological death and rebirth.

Homoeopathy

Homoeopathic remedies work by stimulating the body's own healing power. In 1796 a German doctor, Samuel Hahnemann, discovered a different approach to the cure of the sick, which he called homoeopathy, from the Greek words meaning 'similar suffering'. Like Hippocrates two thousand years earlier he realised that there were two ways of treating ill health; the way of opposites and the way of similars. For example, in the case of insomnia the conventional Western or allopathic way – the way of opposites – is to treat by giving a drug to bring on an artificial sleep. This often involves the use of large or regular doses of drugs that can sometimes cause side effects or addiction. The homoeopathic way – the way of similars – is to give the patient a minute dose of a substance, such as coffee, which in large doses causes sleeplessness in a healthy person. This will enable the patient to sleep naturally. Homoeopathic remedies cannot cause side-effects and you cannot become addicted to them. This is because only a very minute amount of the active ingredient is used in a specially prepared form. The homeopath takes into account your individual characteristics, emotional as well as physical ones.

Homoeopathy is an extremely important alternative to drug treatment and vaccination. It can be used to treat almost any reversible illness in adults, children and animals. Many people do not realise that homoeopathy is also invaluable in helping emotional problems, as well as acute or chronic physical disorders. If you feel emotionally distressed a combination of homoeopathy and counselling or psychotherapy can be just what you need. Homoeopathy is also excellent for children, babies and pregnant women when conventional drugs are not advised.

Huna bodywork

Huna thinking originates in the landscape and world view shared by many island cultures in the Pacific Ocean (Hawaii, Tahiti and the Maori culture in New Zealand). The individual is seen as intimately embedded in relationships with the rest of the world and all these connections are seen as two-way influential. That means a person is seen as both influenced by what is going on around them, in other people and in the natural world, and as influencing it by their own internal and external actions. For example, by thinking of something, or by naming it, we give it strength and help to create it. Individual responsibility for one's own thinking, feeling and doing is stressed, to maximise one's own and others' well-being. Huna assumes that each individual has a conscious, an unconscious and a higher self, and that we can learn to use these aspects of ourselves to achieve personal and social growth and transformation. Huna bodywork derives from the sacred bodywork practised in the temples and as rites of initiation in ancient times. It works with rhythmically induced trance states to achieve an experience of expanded body consciousness and connectedness. PULSING is a modern derivative of this rhythmic expansion of the body and consciousness.

Hydrotherapy

The use of water – solid, (ice), liquid (eg a pool or bath) or vapour – to treat injury, trauma or disease. Physiological responses can be adapted by changing the temperature of the water. Hydrotherapy is one of the oldest types of healing practices, used by Hippocrates in the fifth century BC. The Babylonians, Cretans, Egyptians, Romans and Persians used water baths. To treat disease and for purification Native Americans used vapours in the form of sweat lodges, followed by a plunge in cold water. Nowadays hot baths can, for example, treat arthritis, rheumatism, and gout. Short, cold baths can reduce swelling and pain, and help with fatigue. Vapour and steam baths help the body eliminate toxins through the skin, lungs and kidneys. **Colonic hydrotherapy**, also a treatment used for thousands of years, involves sending warm sterile water into the colon to cleanse out years of accumulated faecal matter, gas, undigested food, parasites, bacteria and toxins.

Iridology

This is a method of assessing states of health and diagnosing physical ills through studying the pupils of the eyes. The condition, pigmentation, structure and marking of the irises are studied in depth. These are unique to each individual. By detecting changes in the eyes, problems can be picked up before they manifest in any of the major systems of the body.

Laughter therapy

Laughter therapy teaches happiness, rather than being a therapy treating problems. At The Happiness Project (see Resources), clients undergo an eight-week Personal Happiness Programme. Laughter is the oldest therapy known to humanity and, like exercise, releases endorphins and encephalins – the body's natural painkillers – into the blood stream. Laughter stimulates and relaxes the muscles, the nervous system, the inner organs, the respiratory system and the heart. Recent research has suggested that laughter helps the immune system, even helping to fight cancer.

Light therapy

Healing through exposure to sunlight or the use of very bright artificial light or ultraviolet light. The latter has helped cure tuberculosis and skin problems such as psoriasis and eczema. Seasonal affective disorder (SAD) and other symptoms such as depression, high blood pressure and insomnia can be helped with bright artificial light. It is possible that it stimulates ovulation and therefore helps with female infertility. (See COLOUR HEALING p. 179)

Magnetic therapy

Often called biomagnetics, this is where specially constructed magnets are used for therapeutic purposes. The magnets stimulate our body's own natural healing ability by increasing blood circulation and thereby bringing increased oxygen to a troubled area in the body. The magnetic polarity that is created dilates blood vessels and increases blood flow to specific areas of tissue. The magnets can be worn inside jewellery or within a wrist band. They can also be placed directly on a site of pain or injury. (Although I know that this therapy does not work for everyone, I have recently started wearing a magnet, called Bioflow, and have found that my yoga practice has quite transformed. A stiffness in my right hip disappeared after forty-eight hours of wearing the magnet on my wrist, and I have considerably more flexibility in all my joints.)

Medical astrology

A form of astrology to help find the root cause of disease. The planets and signs of the zodiac are identified in terms of anatomy and physiology.

Naturopathy

This is the science of healing based on the harmonious relationship between human beings and the earth on which they depend for their sustenance. The primordial requisites of life have to be met in full, and these include adequate rest and sleep; exposure to fresh air, sunshine and warmth; eating wholesome food derived from wholesome soil, providing the body with the nutrients it requires; sufficient exercise; mental and emotional poise to meet the stresses of life; freedom to express opinions; and faith in the capability of the body to renew and repair given appropriate care and time.

Neuro-linguistic programming
An educational and psychological approach to changing behavioural patterns, thoughts, feelings and perceptions in oneself and in communication with others. One of the fundamental beliefs of neuro-linguistic programming (NLP) is that it is easier to change your perception of reality than reality itself. A key word in NLP is 'modelling'; ie the best way to learn a new skill effectively is to do so from somebody who demonstrates it. Modelling means observing very closely how highly skilled people do what they do: what they see, hear, say and feel. NLP teaches techniques to do this. It is not a therapy, but a way of maximising communication. It can therefore be applied in psychotherapy, health care, education, business, performing arts and in any field of work that involves communication.

Nutritional therapy
A health-care system using diet and supplement programmes to correct nutritional deficiencies, combat allergies and help reduce the effects of too much toxicity in the body. The basic constituents of a healthy diet ideally are: plenty of fresh fruits, vegetables and unrefined grains; only a moderate intake of sugar, fat, salt and protein; organically grown foods without the use of artificial fertilisers or pest control; the less processed food the better with the avoidance of potentially harmful preservatives and food additives; variety in the diet, helped by eating locally grown produce in season; preparing food with love and respect and eating it in a relaxed and nourishing environment.

On-site massage
This involves practitioners going to the workplace to treat people in short sessions. It is particularly good for relieving tension and pain in

the back, neck and head. The on-site massage practitioner uses a special kind of seat, which provides support for you to lean into. Various strokes and pressure-point techniques have been adapted to work through the clothes with the body in this relaxed, seated posture.

Orthobionomy

An osteopath and black belt judo instructor in England, Arthur Lincoln Pauls, wanted to work with the body following the line of least resistance. In the early 1970s he combined both Japanese martial arts and osteopathy. Orthobionomy is Greek in origin and loosely means a correct application of the natural laws of life. It is sometimes described as 'homoeopathy of bodywork'.

Pranic healing

Pranic healing utilises prana, the vital energy, or life force, that keeps us alive and healthy. This healing system originates in the Philippines, and it involves cleansing and energising the AURA, and working with the CHAKRAS to aid the ability of the physical body to heal itself. Pranic healers use their hands to scan, or sense, the condition of the aura, chakras and organs. They then use precise energy vibrations, or colours, to help a wide spectrum of ailments. Like all spiritual healing modalities pranic healing can be used as a preventive measure, as there are techniques to boost the immune system and help people to cope with stress.

Psychodrama

This is a form of psychotherapy that uses theatrical techniques practised in a group in a clinical context to help people explore the origins of present-day emotional problems. The client is invited to re-enact an incident — real or imaginary — as if it is a piece of living theatre. She uses others in the group to play roles and then acts as if she is in the original scene. The past is often full of pockets of unfinished business, the emotions from which still underpin and limit our daily functioning. This is archetypal theatre, just as all theatre is potentially a healing medium for the public. By recreating the drama from her own life the client is able to finally deal with painful emotions that she has suppressed.

Psychomotor

An innovative method of psychotherapy and emotional re-education, which began around 1960. It is the work of Al Pesso and Diane Boyden Pesso, and takes place in a controlled setting on a symbolic level. The episodes of therapeutic work are called structures. This work is often in groups and usually includes the client choosing another individual or an object to play a role of a significant person in her life (past or present). Techniques called positive or negative accommodation are used. For example, in positive accommodation the client asks for actions or messages she would like to hear from the role player. It may be something she needed to hear as a child from a parent, such as 'you are lovable'. One aim of negative accommodation is to help the client express anger. The person playing the role makes a sound or action that is congruent with the amount of anger expressed by the client. The purpose of the work is to help the client resolve past conflicts and satisfy previously unmet needs. Past emotional injuries can be healed and new parts of the self are enabled to emerge and become integrated into the functioning of the person.

My personal experience of this work is that it was deeply healing and satisfying; changes that freed me and made me feel more fully myself took place within my physical body.

Psychosynthesis

This is a form of psychotherapy that embraces the soul, the imagination and the will in its theories. It was developed by Roberto Assagioli during the first part of the twentieth century. Meditation and visualisation are two of its core methods.

RADIX®

RADIX® was originated by Charles Kelley and employs techniques from GESTALT THERAPY, BIO-ENERGETICS, BATES METHOD OF VISION TRAINING and ERIKSONIAN HYPNOTHERAPY. It is a NEO-REICHIAN educational model through which people learn how to experience, express and manage feelings that are trapped in deep body tissues. Two central ideas are safety and exploration. Exploration grows out of the sense of safety created by a trusting, comfortable environment, so that individuals can go into the arena of the somatic (or body) experience of emotions.

SHEN

Developed by an American scientist called Richard Pavek in the 1980s, SHEN stands for specific human energy nexus. The aim of this therapy is physical and emotional release. The practitioner works in a carefully planned pattern, gently resting the hands on the client's clothed body. Like SUBTLE ENERGY HEALING it recognises the relationship between physical symptoms and particular emotions. For example, contracted emotions can lead to heart failure; anger, fear or anxiety manifest in the solar plexus and can result in digestive disorders; guilt, shame, security, confidence and helplessness have their roots in the navel/pubic regions and so on.

The Silva Method

This is a 'mind–control' method, which teaches you how to function with greater self-awareness and self-control by entering an inner, conscious brain level called the alpha state. Studies show that this deeply meditative state stimulates the memory, and can accelerate learning, improve intuition and enhance creativity.

Somatic emotional therapy

This psychotherapeutic approach has been developed by Stanley Keleman and is based on his theoretical concepts of formative psychology. The director of the Centre for Energetic Studies in Berkeley, California, he is a pioneer in the field of connections between anatomy and feeling. It is through our anatomy, our physical body, that we experience emotion. Traditional anatomy shows two-dimensional images that leave out the most important element: our emotional life. At the same time psychology, which is committed to the study of emotion, lacks anatomical understanding. To Keleman consciousness is the body. From the beginning of life, molecules and cells organise into clusters that further organise as layers, tubes, tunnels and pouches, giving structure to liquid life and setting the stage for human consciousness. We form our shape. This shape is changed by how we respond emotionally to those around us and the events of our lives, for example, the effects of love, disappointments, insults, assaults, and all the challenges and stresses of existence. Keleman's work is a major influence in body psychotherapy.

Transcendental Meditation

Meditation is used to focus the mind and to reach a state of inner tranquillity and increased awareness. During the process of relaxation and concentration in meditation, breathing, brain activity and the heart and pulse rate slow down. This enables the body to return to a state of homeostasis. Transcendental Meditation was taught in the 1960s by Maharishi Mahesh Yogi. It involves a commitment to regular meditation practice and involves repeating, or chanting, a mantra. Mantras are sacred words or phrases. Meditation has been found to help alleviate a wide range of physical and emotional problems, from acute anxiety, asthma and high blood pressure to premenstrual syndrome (PMS), menopausal symptoms and migraine. It is always best to learn to meditate with a teacher.

Notes

Introduction

1. The sacrum is a wedge-shaped bone formed by the fusion of five vertebrae below the lumbar vertebrae towards the base of the spine. It forms part of the back of the wall of the pelvis.

Chapter One

The Holistic Approach

1. Dr Christiane Northrup, *Women's Bodies Women's Wisdom*, Piatkus, 1995, p.12
2. Lynne McTaggart, *What Doctors Don't Tell You*, Thorsons, 1996, back cover
3. Ted Kaptchuk, *Chinese Medicine; The Web That Has No Weaver*, Rider & Co, 1983, p.2
4. Sarah Cant and Ursula Sharma, eds, *Complementary and Alternative Medicines: Knowledge in Practice*, Free Association Books, 1996, Introduction
5. Ibid
6. Daniel Garger, 'Science and Certainty in Descartes' in Michael Hooker, ed, *Descartes*, Johns Hopkins University Press, 1978, quoted in Beinfield and Korngold, eds, *Between Heaven and Earth; A Guide to Chinese Medicine*, Ballantine Books, 1991, p.17
7. Fred Sommers, 'Dualism in Descartes: The Logical Ground' in Michael Hooker, ed, *Descartes*, Johns Hopkins University Press, 1979

8. Barbara Ann Brennan, *Hands of Light*, Bantam Books, 1987, p.22

9. Ibid, p.23

10. Ibid, p.25

11. Fritjof Capra, *The Tao of Physics*, Fontana/Collins, 1975, p.23

12. Ashley Montagu, *Touching: The Human Significance of the Skin*, Harper & Row, 1971, 1997, p.261

13. Alexander Lowen, *The Betrayal of the Body*, pp.2–3

14. Novalis, quoted in Thomas Carlyle, *Miscellaneous Essays*, volume II

Chapter Two

The Meaning of Illness

1. Ken Wilber, *Grace and Grit*, Gill and Macmillan, 1991, p.40

2. Caroline Myss, *Anatomy of the Spirit*, Bantam, 1997, p.48

3. Lesley Doyal, *What Makes Women Sick*, Macmillan Publishing Ltd, 1995, p.7

4. Dr Christiane Northrup, *Women's Bodies Women's Wisdom*, Introduction

5. Ibid, p.4

6. Myss, op cit, p.47

7. McTaggart, op cit, p.xxviii

8. The brain stem, at the base of the brain, is at the beginning of the spinal column.

9. Arachnoiditis is inflammation of one of the coverings round the brain.

10. Stephen Levine, *Healing into Life and Death*, Gateway Books, 1989, 1995, p.5

11. Myss, op cit, p.57

12. For example, the humoral pathological blood test and the work of Prof D Schweitzer at The Essential Health Clinic, 32 Notting Hill Gate, London W11 3HX, tel. 020 7221 6932, http:www.davidschweitzer.com

13. Bernie Segal, *Love, Medicine and Miracles*, Arrow Books, 1988, p.69

14. Wayne W Dyer, *Manifest Your Destiny*, Thorsons, 1998, p.57

15. Ibid, p.57

16. Deepak Chopra, *The Seven Spiritual Laws of Success*, Bantam Books, 1996, p.70

17. The left and right sides of the brain refer to a very simplistic distinction between types of brain function. The left side, which controls the right side of the body, is to do with logical, cause and effect, linear thinking. The right side, which controls the left side of the body, is to do with creative, intuitive, 'holistic' thinking. Sometimes masculine qualities are associated with the left and feminine the right.

Chapter Three

Touch and Contact

1. Bernd Eiden, 'The Use of Touch in Psychotherapy', *Self and Society*, Vol 26, No 2, May 1998, pp.3–8

2. Kate Williams, 'Recognising the Importance of Being Touched', unpublished paper, May 1998

3. Ashley Montagu, *Touching, The Human Significance of the Skin*, Harper & Row, 1971, p.100

4. MDS Ainsworth, *Infancy in Uganda*, Johns Hopkins University Press, 1967, p.451

5. R James de Boer, *The Netsilik Eskimo and the Origin of Human Behaviour*, 1969, p.8, in Ashley Montagu, *Touching, The Human Significance of the Skin*, p.297

6. O Schaeffer, 'When the Eskimo Comes to Town', *Nutrition Today*, November 1971, pp.8–16, in *Touching, The Human Significance of the Skin*, Harper & Row, 1971

7. Montagu, op cit, pp.322–3

Chapter Four

Finding a Practitioner or Therapist

1. Tittany Field, Maria Hernandex-Reif, Sybil Hart, Olga Quintino, Levelle Dros, Tory Feld, 'Effects of sexual abuse are lessened by

massage therapy', in *Journal of Bodywork and Movement Therapies*, January 1997

2. The LETS scheme is based on exchanging skills within local communities. Money is not used. Skills are given a value and this forms a 'currency' in the form of pledges.

Chapter Five

The Massage Therapies

1. For codes of ethics and practice and training information refer to British Massage Council (see Resources).

2. Jane Alexander, *Supertherapies*, Bantam Books, 1996, p.147

3. Two examples of charitable organisations where complementary therapies are used in the management of cancer are: Cancer Care, North Lancs & South Lakeland Support & Information Service, Slynedales, Lancaster Road, Lancaster, tel: 01524 381820; and Wandsworth Cancer Support Centre, PO Box 17, 20-22 York Road, London SW11 3QE, tel: 0207 924 3924.

4. The Association of Chartered Physiotherapists in Bio-Energy Therapies (see Resources).

5. Mel Cash, *Sports and Remedial Massage Therapy*, Ebury Press, 1996, p.59

6. Isotonic exercise involves movement of the joints and muscles; as in weight lifting or with the variable resistance machines now popular in gyms or health clubs. Isometric exercise involves little or no movement. The muscle is merely contracted – usually against an opposing force – as in the MUSCLE ENERGY TECHNIQUE.

7. See Selected Reading and Resources for further information, especially Patricia Davis, *Aromatherapy A–Z*, CW Daniel Co Ltd, 1988; and Jane Dye, *Aromatherapy for Women and Children*, CW Daniel Co Ltd, 1992

8. See Allison England, *Aromatherapy for Mother and Baby*, Vermillion, 1993

9. E Burns and C Blamey, 'Soothing Scents in Childbirth', *International Journal of Aromatherapy*, 6, 24–8, 1994, in Stephen Fulder,

Handbook of Alternative and Complementary Medicine, Vermilion, 1996, p.228

Chapter Six

Manipulation Therapies and Postural Education
1. Tingling fingers can often be caused by subluxation of the neck vertebrae.
2. Hilary Dewey 'Osteopathy', in *Part 2, A–Z of Complementary Therapies in Medical Marriage*, p.378. Hilary Dewey was a qualified nurse and midwife before becoming an osteopath.
3. Kathy Webster Bates, 'Rolfing; Structural Integration', in *Medical Marriage*, p.461
4. Rosemary Feitis in *Bone, Breath and Gesture*, Don Hanson Johnson, ed, North Atlantic Books, 1995, p.163, referring to Ida Rolf's article 'Gravity: an Unexplored Factor in a More Human Use of Human Beings' in *Systematics*, Vol 1, No. 1, June 1963
5. FM Alexander, 'Notes of Instruction', in Edward Maisel, *Essential Writings of FM Alexander*

Chapter Seven

Zones, Meridians and Pressure Point Therapies
1. Ted Kaptchuk, *Chinese Medicine; The Web That Has No Weaver*, Rider & Co, 1983, p.2
2. Beinfeld and Korngold, eds, *Between Heaven and Earth; A Guide to Chinese Medicine*, Ballantine Books, 1991, p.17
3. From *Ne Jing*, a medical classic written in the second century BC.
4. Myofascial refers to fascia that covers muscle. Fascia is the connective tissue found throughout the body.
5. A sebaceous cyst is a benign, harmless growth under the skin, usually on the scalp, face, ears and genitals, where the release of sebum is blocked. They only need treatment if they become large or painful.
6. Ray Ridolfe and Susanne Franzen, *Shiatsu for Women*, p.3

7. B Harris and R Lewis, *International Journal of Alternative and Complementary Medicine*, 1995, in Stephen Fulder, *The Handbook of Alternative and Complementary Medicine*
8. Nicola Hall, *Reflexology for Women*, Thorsons, 1994 p.62
9. Ibid, p.67
10. Jane Alexander quoting Dr Stone in *Supertherapies*, p.286
11. Rosamund Webster, 'Polarity Therapy', in *Medical Marriage*, p.392
12. Maggie La Tourelle with Anthea Courtenay, *Principles of Kinesiology*, Thorsons, 1997, p.5
13. John Thie is the originator of *Touch for Health*. Lori Forsyth quotes him in 'Kinesiology', *Medical Marriage*, p.307
14. Ibid, Forsyth, p.307
15. Ibid, Forsyth, p.312

Chapter Eight

The Metaphysical Therapies
1. Note: For an excellent source of scientific evidence for a number of forms of spiritual healing read Dr Daniel Benor, *Healing Research*, Helix Editions Ltd, Centrepoint, Chapel Square, Deddington, Oxfordshire, 1993
2. Spiritualism is the belief in life after death, and that dead people can be contacted and communicated with through a medium.
3. Anthea Courtenay, *Healing Now*, Dent & Sons Ltd, 1991, p.1
4. You can often have your aura photographed at Mind, Body and Spirit, or Complementary Health Exhibitions that happen in most cities and large towns regularly. I discovered a shop in Brighton, Sussex that has an aura camera. You can be photographed in the shop. They also hire out a camera with operator and analyst. They now have a second camera. Here the image is a moving one. You can see your body, aura and chakras on a computer monitor. With either camera you can have a before and after picture, and see what changes have occurred by receiving healing or doing meditation or some other energy balancing activity. Contact: Winfalcon's Wholistic Shop and Healing Centre, 28 Ship Street, Brighton, Sussex BN1 1AD, tel:

01273 728997; winfalcon@dial.pipex.com

5. Barbara Ann Brennan, op cit. References to the aura are made throughout the book.

6. Plasma is the fluid portion of the blood or lymph.

7. Metabolism means the sum of all the physical and chemical processes to sustain life, and the transformation by which energy (from a mechanical point of view) is made available to the body.

8. The *Oxford English Dictionary* defines placebo as 'a substance or procedure which a patient accepts as a medicine or therapy activity for his condition or is prescribed in the belief that it has no such activity.' The placebo effect is 'a beneficial (or adverse) effect produced by a placebo that cannot be attributed to the nature of the placebo.'

9. *American Journal of Nursing*, quoted on inside cover of Dolores Krieger, *Accepting Your Power to Heal*, Bear & Co. Publishing, 1993.

10. Jean Sayre Adams, 'Therapeutic Touch; Principles and Practice', in *Complementary Therapies in Medicine*, 1993, 1, pp.96–9

11. Ibid, pp.96–9

12. Jane Alexander, *Supertherapies*, p.328

13. Ibid, p.330

14. See the therapeutic uses of colour, pp. 180–8

15. Ohms are units of electrical resistance. They measure the work that an electrical charge has to do to move through a material (ie body tissue). Disease changes the resistance of body tissue.

16. Theo Gimbel, *Healing with Colour*, Gaia Books Ltd, 1994, p.20

17. Ibid, p.12

18. Solarized water is water that has been surrounded with a coloured filter and placed in sunlight for a couple of hours. The colours of light are thought to affect the water's molecules, giving them the energy of the colour they receive. You slowly drink the water to get the benefits.

19. Kate Williams is a massage practitioner, healer and psychotherapist. She is co-principal of The Rowan School of Healing and Personal Development.

20. Olivea Dewhurst-Maddock, *Healing with Sound*, p.11

21. Lawrence Buchan, 'Sound Therapy', in *Medical Marriage*, p.482

22. Dewhurst-Maddock, op cit, p.13

23. Barbara Ann Brennan, op cit, p.241
24. Fabien Maman, *Technique of Pure Sound: Healing Mind, Body and Spirit*, Caduceus, 1988, 5, pp.5–6
25. Lawrence Buchan, 'Sound Therapy', in *Medical Marriage*, p.486

Chapter Nine

Body Psychotherapy, Including Rebirthing and Hypnotherapy

1. See the UK Council for Psychotherapy list of registered centres and psychotherapists, Humanistic and Integrative Section. UKCP, 167–169 Great Portland Street, London W1N 5FB, tel: 0171 436 3002.
2. Stanley Kelemen, *Your Body Speaks Its Mind*, Center Press, p. 13
3. Chiron Centre web site http://www.chiron.org (see Resources)
4. Bernd Eiden, 'Reich's Legacy', in *Counselling News – the voice of counselling training*, January 1999
5. Richard Hoff, *Overview of Reichian Therapy*, p.338 in *The New Holistic Health Handbook*, Berkeley Holistic Health Center, The Stephen Grene Press, 1985
6. Elaine Stillerman, *The Encyclopaedia of Bodywork*, p.35
7. Elaine Stillerman, *The Encyclopaedia of Bodywork*, p. 106
8. Gill Westland, in *Complementary Therapies in Nursery and Midwifery*
9. Ibid
10. Frederich S Perls, *In and Out the Garbage Pail*, Real People Press, 1966
11. Jennifer MacKewn, 'Modern Gestalt – an Integrative and Ethical Approach to Counselling and Psychotherapy', *Counselling*, May 1994
12. Sheila Ernst and Lucy Goodison, 'In Our Own Hands', p.59
13. John O Stevens, *Awareness*, p.83
14. Michael Sky, *Breathing: Expanding your Power and Energy*, p126
15. Bernadette Riley, 'Breathing', in *Cahoots*, issue 57
16. Gunnel Minnet, *Breath and Spirit*, p.20
17. Anna Bondizio, 'Rebirthing', *Medical Marriage*, p.433. Also refer to Chapter 3, *Touch and Contact*

18. Stephen Fulder, *The Handbook of Alternative and Complementary Medicine*, p.211
19. R Asher, 'Respectable Hypnosis', *British Medical Association Journal*, 1, 309–13, 1956

Chapter Ten

Energy Movement Systems

1. Lucy Lidell with Narayani and Giris Rainovitch, *The Book of Yoga*, Ebury Press, 1983, p.15
2. TKV Desikachar, *Patanjali's Yogasutras*, Ch 1, Yogasutras, sutra (ie verse) No 2
3. Ibid, Ch 2, sutra 29
4. Lucy Lidell *et al*, *The Book of Yoga*
5. In the CHAKRA system this point, around one and a half to two inches below the navel, is referred to as the hara or sacral centre (see Chapter 8)
6. Elaine Stillerman, *The Encyclopedia of Bodywork*, p.229
7. ME is short for Myalgic Encephalomyelitis, sometimes called post-viral syndrome. It is characterised by a multitude of symptoms and signs, the most common being severe fatigue precipitated by minimal exertion and not relieved by rest, generalised aches and pains, depression, and problems adjusting to changes in temperature. At present it remains poorly understood.
8. Raynaud's disease is defined as intermittent, cold-precipitated symmetrical attacks of pallor and/or blueness (called cyanosis) of the digits without any evidence of obstructive arterial disease (*Basic Clinical Science* by Dr Nic Rowley).
9. Lynne Robinson and Gordon Thomas, *Body Control, The Pilates Way*, p.11
10. Ibid, p.12
11. Barbara Barnes, Feldenkrais teacher, *Positive Living Magazine*, Issue 23, 1997
12. Chantal Kickz, 'Feldenkrais Method', *Medical Marriage*, p.233
13. Neshama Franklin, *The New Holistic Health Handbook*, p.333

14. Rosa Shreeves, *Imaginary Dances*, Wardlock Educational Co Ltd, 1998. Rosa is a dance artist and therapist, and believes in the self-healing and expressive power of movement and the creative arts.

15. Katya Bloom and Rosa Shreeves, *Moves*, Harwood Academic Publishers, 1998, Introduction. A source book of ideas for body awareness and creative movement.

16. Ibid

17. Anita Green, 'Dancing Towards Health', *Nursing Times*, Sept 13, Vol 85, No 37, 1989

Chapter Eleven

Convergence Therapies

1. Marion Rosen quoted in Elaine Loomis Mayland, *The Rosen Method*, 1984, p.13

2. cf Freud, Chapter 9

3. Elaine Loomis Mayland, op cit, p.15

4. Ibid, p.16

5. Paul Cohen, 'Zero Balancing', *Positive Health*, July 1998

6. Jane Alexander, article in the *Daily Mail*, 27.1.96

7. Deane Juhan, Trager practitioner and instructor, author of *Job's Body: A Handbook for Bodywork*.

8. Gaston Saint-Pierre and Debbie Boater, *The Metamorphic Technique*, p.16

9. Guy Gladstone, 'Pulsing – Massage in Motion: Energy and Character', *The Journal of Biosynthesis*, Vol 16, No 2, August 1985

10. Ashley Montagu, op cit, p.128

Selected Reading

Reference Books

Jack Angelo, *Your Healing Power; A Comprehensive Guide to Channelling Your Healing Energies*, Piatkus, London, 1995

Jane Alexander, *Supertherapies; New Ways to Rejuvenate Body, Mind and Spirit*, Bantam Books, London, 1996

Ellen Bass and Laura Davis, *The Courage to Heal; A Guide for Women Survivors of Child Sexual Abuse*, Harper & Row Publishers, New York, 1988; Mandarin, London, 1990

Beinfield and Korngold, *Between Heaven and Earth; A Guide to Chinese Medicine*, Ballantine Books, New York, 1991

Dr Daniel Benor, *Healing Research; Holistic Energy Medicine and Spirituality*, Helix Editions Ltd, Deddington, Oxfordshire, 1993

Katya Bloom and Rosa Shreeves, *Moves; A Sourcebook of Ideas for Body Awareness, and Creative Movement*, Harwood Academic Publishers, UK, 1998

The Boston Women's Health Book Collective, *Our Bodies, Ourselves for the New Century*, Touchstone, 1999

Gil Boyne, *Transforming Therapy; A New Approach to Hypnotherapy*, Westwood Publishing Co Inc, Glendale, CA, 1989

Barbara Ann Brennan, *Hands of Light; A Guide to Healing Through the Human Energy Field*, Bantam Books, USA and Canada, 1987

Elisabeth Brooke, *Women Healers Through History*, The Women's Press, London, 1992

Dr Craig Brown, *Optimum Healing; A Life-Changing Approach to Achieving Good Health*, Rider, London, 1998

Loulou Brown, *Alternative Medicine; Teach Yourself Books*, Hodder & Stoughton, London, 1999

Eve Cameron and Karena Callen, *Cosmopolitan; One-to-one Massage; Expert Techniques to Relax and Stimulate*, Ebury Press, London, 1993

Sarah Cant and Ursula Sharma, eds, *Complementary and Alternative Medicines; Knowledge in Practice*, Free Association Books Ltd, London and New York, 1996

Mel Cash, *Sports and Remedial Massage Therapy*, Ebury Press, London, 1996

Deepak Chopra, *Quantum Healing; Exploring the Frontiers of Mind/Body Medicine*, Bantam, New York & Toronto, 1989

Anthea Courtenay, *Healing Now*, Dent & Sons Ltd, London, 1991 (out of print)

Dr Brenda Davies, *Rainbow Journey; Seven Steps to Self Healing*, Hodder & Stoughton, London, 1998

Drs Brenda Davies and Hilary Jones, *Total Well-Being; The Whole Treatment for the Whole You*, Hodder & Stoughton, London, 1999

Patricia Davis, *Aromatherapy; An A–Z*, CW Daniel Co Ltd, Saffron Walden, England, 1988

Olivea Dewhurst-Maddock, *Healing with Sound*, Gaia Books Limited, London, 1993, new edition 1997

Lesley Doyal, *What Makes Women Sick; Gender and the Political Economy of Health*, Macmillan Publishing Ltd, London, 1995

Jane Dye, *Aromatherapy for Women and Children*, CW Daniel Co Ltd, Saffron Walden, England, 1992

Dave Elman, *Hypnotherapy*, Westwood Publishing Co Inc, Glendale, CA, 1970

Sheila Ernst and Lucy Goodison, *In Our Own Hands; A Book of Self-Help Therapy*, The Women's Press, London 1981, 1982, 1984, 1985

Dr Cornelia Featherstone and Lori Forsyth, *Medical Marriage; The New Partnership between Orthodox and Complementary Medicine*, Findhorn Press, Scotland, 1997

Marilyn Ferguson, *The Aquarian Conspiracy*, Granada Publishing Ltd, London, 1982

Stephen Fulder, *The Handbook of Alternative and Complementary Medicine; The Essential Health Companion*, Vermilion, London 1996

Richard Gerber MD, *Vibrational Medicine; New Choices for Healing Ourselves*, Bear & Company, Sante Fe, New Mexico, 1988

Michael Gienger, *Crystal Power, Crystal Healing; The Complete Handbook*, Blandford, London, 1998

Theo Gimbel, *Healing with Colour*, Gaia Books Limited, London, 1994

Nicola Hall, *Reflexology for Women; Restore Harmony and Balance Through Precise Massaging Techniques*, Thorsons, London, 1994

Dr Hilary Jones, *Doctor, What's The Alternative?; Everything You Need to Know about Complementary Therapy*, Hodder & Stoughton, London, 1998

Ted J Kaptchuk, *Chinese Medicine; The Web That Has No Weaver*, Rider & Co, 1983

Stanley Keleman, *Emotional Anatomy*, Center Press, Berkeley, CA, 1985

Stanley Keleman, *Love*, Center Press, Berkeley, CA, 1994

Stanley Keleman, *Your Body Speaks Its Mind*, Center Press, Berkeley, CA, 1981

Leslie Kenton, *Passage to Power; Natural Menopause Revolution*, Ebury Press, London, 1995

Dolores Krieger, *Accepting Your Power to Heal; The Personal Practice of Therapeutic Touch*, Bear & Company, Sante Fe, New Mexico, 1993

Maggie La Tourelle with Anthea Courtenay, *Principles of Kinesiology; The Only Introduction You'll Ever Need*, Thorsons, London, 1997

Stephen Levine, *Healing Into Life and Death*, Gateway Books, Bath, England 1997

Lucinda Lidell, *The Book of Massage; The Complete Step-to-Step Guide to Eastern and Western Techniques*, Ebury Press, London, 1984

Brenda Mallon, *Creative Visualization with Colour; Healing Your Life with the Power of Colour*, Element, Shaftesbury, 1999

Lynne McTaggart, *What Doctors Don't Tell You; The Truth about the Dangers of Modern Medicine*, Thorsons, London, 1996

Gunnel Minett, *Breath and Spirit; Rebirthing as a Healing Technique*, The Aquarian Press, London, 1994

Ashley Montagu, *Touching: The Human Significance of the Skin*, Harper & Row, New York, 1971, 1978, 1986, 1997

Jim Morningstar, *Breathing in Light and Love; Your Call to Breath and Body Mastery*, Transformations Incorporated, US, 1994

Caroline Myss, *Anatomy of the Spirit; The Seven Stages of Power and Healing*, Bantam Books, London, 1996

Dr Christiane Northrup, *Women's Bodies Women's Wisdom; The Complete Guide to Women's Health and Wellbeing*, Piatkus, London, 1995

Frederich S Perls, *In and Out of the Garbage Pail!*, Real People Press, 1996

Ray Ridolfe and Susanne Franzen, *Shiatsu for Women*, Thorsons, London, 1996

Lynne Robinson and Gordon Thomson, *Body Control; The Pilates Way*, Boxtree, London, 1997

Peter Rutter MD, *Sex in the Forbidden Zone; When Men in Power – Therapists, Doctors, Clergy, Teachers and Others – Betray Women's Trust*, Mandala Unwin Paperbacks, London, 1990

Gaston Saint-Pierre and Debbie Boater, *The Metamorphic Technique, Principles and Practice*, Element Books Ltd, Shaftesbury, England, 1985

Liz Simpson, *The Book of Crystal Healing*, Gaia Books Limited, London, 1997

Michael Sky, *Breathing; Expanding your Power and Energy*, Bear and Co, Santa Fe, New Mexico, 1990

Diane Stein, *Essential Reiki; A Complete Guide to an Ancient Healing Art*, The Crossing Press Inc, Freedom, CA, 4th printing 1996

John O Stevens, *Awareness; Exploring, Experimenting, Experiencing*, Real People Press, Moab, Utah, US, 1971; Eden Grove Editions, London 1989

Maryon Stewart and Dr Alan Stewart, *Every Woman's Health Guide; The Women's Nutritional Advisory Service Handbook for Drug-Free Health*, Headline, London, 1997

Elaine Stillerman, *The Encyclopaedia of Bodywork; From Acupressure to Zone Therapy*, Facts on File, Inc, New York, 1996

Charles Tebbetts, *Miracles on Demand; The Radical Short-Term Hypnotherapy*, The Hypnotism Training Institute of Washington, Edmonds, WA, 1985

Milton Trager with Cathy Hammond, *Movement as a Way to Agelessness; A Guide to Trager Mentastics*, Station Hill Press, 1987, 1995

Michael Tse, *Qigong for Health and Vitality*, Piatkus Books, London, 1995

Peter Walker, *Baby Massage; A Practical Guide to Massaging and Movement for Babies and Infants*, Piatkus, London, 1995

Ouida West, *The Magic of Massage; A New and Holistic Approach*, Century Publishing, London, 1983

Ruth White, *Working with Your Chakras*, Piatkus, London, 1993

Ken Wilber, *Grace and Grit; Spirituality and Healing in the Life and Death of Treya Killam Wilber*, Gill & Macmillan, Boston, US, 1991

Magazines

Caduceus
38 Russell Terrace
Leamington Spa
Warwickshire CV31 1HE
tel: 01926 451897

Human Potential Magazine
5 Layton Road
Islington
London N1
tel: 020 7354 5793

Kindred Spirit
Foxhole
Dartington
Totnes
Devon TQ9 6EB
tel: 01803 866686
fax: 01803 866591

editors@kindredspirit.co.uk
http://www.kindredspirit.co.uk

Positive Health
Positive Health Publications Ltd
51 Queens Square
Bristol BS1 4LJ
tel: 0117 983 8851
fax: 0117 908 0097
mike@positive.u.et.com
sandra@positive.u.net.com
http://www.positivehealth.com
00117 983 8851

Proof!
4 Wallace Road
London N1 2PG
tel: 020 7354 4592
fax: 020 7354 8907
wddty@zoo.co.uk

Resources

The following pages contain organisations relevant to the therapies described in the book and in the chapter order in which they are described. If you want to find out about a particular organisation that is not listed here, please contact one of the general organisations, which are listed first. Australia, New Zealand and US have been included, although in less detail than the UK list. Details of specific therapies in these countries should be available via the relevant national organisation of the country concerned, or a national or specific UK organisation.

UK

National Organisations

The Association of Chartered
Physiotherapists in Bio-Energy
Therapies
Secretary: Rowena Cook
2 Preston Paddock
Rustington
Sussex BN16 2AA

British Complementary
Medicine Association
33 Imperial Square
Cheltenham
Gloucestershire GL50 1QZ
fax: 01242 227765

Council for Complementary
and Alternative Medicine
Park House
206-208 Latimer Road

London W10 6RE
tel: 020 8968 3862

The Disability Foundation
Edgware Community Hospital
Edgware Road
Edgware
Middlesex HA8 OAD
tel: 020 8952 5410
fax: 020 8952 5412
info@the-disability-
foundation.org.uk
www.the-disability-
foundation.org.uk

Guild of Complementary
Practitioners
Liddell House
Liddell Close
Finchampstead
Berkshire G40 4NS
tel: 0118 973 5757
fax: 0118 973 5767

Pain Concern UK
PO Box 318
Canterbury
Kent CT4 5DP
tel: 01227 712183

Research Council for
Complementary Medicine
60 Great Ormond Street
London WC1N 3JF
tel: 020 7833 8897
fax: 020 7278 7412
rccm@gn.apc.org

Spinal Injuries Association
76 St James's Lane
London N10 3DF
tel: 020 8444 2121
fax: 020 8444 3767
sia@spinali.demon.co.uk
jgrweb.com/sia/

Women's Health
A Resource and Information
Centre
52 Featherstone Street
London EC1Y 8RT
tel: 0207 251 6580

**Massage Therapies and
Aromatherapy**

British Massage Therapy
Council
2 Layer Gardens
London W3 9PR
tel: 020 8992 2554

Scottish Massage Therapists
Organization
70 Lochside Road
Denmore Park
Bridge of Don
Aberdeen AB23 8QW
tel: 01224 822956

Indian Head Massage
c/o Mr Narendra Mehta
136 Holloway Road
London N7 8DD
tel: 020 7607 3331
fax: 020 7607 4228

The International Association
for Infant Massage
72 Coningsworth Road
Carlton
Nottingham NG4 3SJ
tel: 0115 9870655

International Federation of
Aromatherapists
Stamford House
2-4 Chiswick High Road
London W4 1TH
tel: 020 8742 2605

International Society of
Professional Aromatherapists
ISPA House
82 Ashby Road
Hinkley
Leicestershire LE10 1SN
tel: 01455 637 987

The Manipulation Therapies and Postural Education

General Osteopathic Council
Premier House
10 Greycoat Place
London SW1P 1SB
tel: 020 7799 2442
fax: 020 7799 2332
gosc@osteopathy.org.uk

The Sutherland Society
(to find a local cranial
osteopath)
c/o The Crouch End Natural
Health Clinic
170 Weston Park
London N8 9PN
tel: 020 8341 9800
cranial.net@virgin.net
vzone.virgin.net/big.phil

British Chiropractic Association
Blagrave House
17 Blagrave Stret
Reading RG1 1QB
tel: 01189 505950
fax: 01189 588946

McTimoney Chiropractic
Association
21 High Street
Eynsham
Oxford OX8 1HE
tel: 01865 880974
fax: 01865 880975

Society of Teachers of the
Alexander Technique
20 London House
266 Fulham Road
London SW10 9EL
tel: 020 7351 0828
fax: 020 7352 1556

Zones, Meridians and Pressure Point Therapies

Association of Chinese
Acupuncture
Prospect House
2 Grove Lane
Retford
Nottinghamshire
DN22 6NA
tel: 01777 704411
fax: 01777 704411

British Acupuncture Council
63 Jeddo Road
London W12 9HJ
tel: 020 8735 0400
fax: 020 8735 0404
www.acupuncture.org.uk

British Medical Acupuncture
Society
Newton House
Newton Lane
Whitley
Warrington
Cheshire WA4 4JA
tel: 01925 730727
fax: 01925 730492

Applied Kinesiology:
Integrated Practitioner Training
70a Caversham Road
Kentish Town
London NW5 2DS
tel: 020 7485 4215

Kinesiology Foundation
PO Box 7891
London SW19 1ZB
tel: 020 8545 1255

British Polarity Council
Monomonk House
27 Old Gloucester Street
London WC1N 3XX
tel: 01483 417714

The Shiatsu Society
Barber House
Storeys Bar Road
Fengate
Peterborough, PE1 5YS
tel: 01733 758341

Metaphysical Therapies

The Association for Therapeutic
Healers
79 Brixton Hill
London SW2 1JE
tel: 07074 222284

British Alliance of Healing
Associations
3 Sandy Lane
Gisleham

Lowestoft
Suffolk NR33 8EQ
tel: 01502 742224

British Alliance of Healing
Organisations
23 Nutcroft Grove
Fetcham
Leatherhead
Surrey KT22 9LA
tel: 01372 373241

The British Association of
Therapeutic Touch
Highland Hall
Renwick
Penrith
Cumbria CA10 1JL
tel: 01768 898375

Confederation of Healing
Organisations
The Red and White House
113 High Street
Berkhamstead
Herts HP4 2DJ
tel: 01442 870660

Living Magically
Fisher Beck Mill
Old Lake Road
Ambleside
Cumbria LA22 0DH
tel: 015394 31943
fax: 015394 31946
info@livingmagically.co.uk
www.livingmagically.co.uk

The National Federation of
Spiritual Healers
Old Manor Farm Studio
Church Street
Sunbury on Thames
Middlesex TW16 6RG
tel: 01932 783164
fax: 01932 779647
office@nfsh.org.uk

The Radionic Association
Baerlein House
Goose Green
Deddington
Banbury
Oxon OX15 OSX
tel: 01869 338 852

Reiki Association
Cornbrook Bridge House
Clee Hill
Ludlow
Shropshire SY8 3QQ
tel: 01584 891197

The Rowan School for Healing
and Personal Growth
126 Chase Way
Southgate
London N14 5DH
tel: 020 8368 9868
fax: 020 8368 8772
rowan.school@virgin.net

Affiliation of Crystal Healing
Organisations
PO Box 344

Manchester M60 2EZ
tel: 0161 278 0096

Hygeia Studios
Colour Therapy
Brook House
Avening
Tetbury
Gloucestershire GL8 8NS
tel: 01453 832150

School of Living Light
47 Aldrath Road
Haddenham
Cambridgeshire CB6 3PW
tel: 01353 741760
fax: 01353 741782

Body Psychotherapy, including Rebirthing and Hypnotherapy

The Association of Holistic
Biodynamic Massage Therapists
(AHBMT)
20 Oak Drive
Larkfield
Aylesford
Kent ME20 6NU
tel/fax: 01732 875 605

The Cambridge Body
Psychotherapy Centre
28 Ditton Walk
Cambridge CP5 8QE
tel: 01223 416 166

The Chiron Centre for Body
Psychotherapy
26 Eaton Rise
Ealing
London W5 2ER
tel: 020 8997 5219

European Association for Body-
Psychotherapy
Secretariat
Avenue Pictet-de-
Rochemont 7
CH-1207 Geneva,
Switzerland

Hakomi Therapy
hakomiuk@fastnet.co.uk

The Open Centre
188 Old Street
London EC1V 9FR
tel: 020 7272 6672

Spectrum
Centre for Humanistic and
Integrative Psychotherapy
7 Endymion Road
London N4 1EE
tel: 020 8341 2277

Spectrum Incest Intervention
Project
(psychotherapy for victims,
survivors and perpetrators of
sexual abuse and their families)
7 Endymion Road
London N4 1EE
tel: 020 8348 0196

The British Rebirth Society
c/o Bernadette Riley
Lawnswood
22 Rossall Road
Lytham St Annes
Lancs. FY8 4ES
tel: 01253 739107

National Register of
Hypnotherapists and
Psychotherapists
12 Cross Street
Nelson
Lancashire BB9 7EN
tel: 01282 699378
fax: 01282 698633

The Women's Therapy Centre
10 Manor Gardens
London N7 6JS
tel: 020 7263 6200

Movement Therapies

Association for Dance
Movement Therapy
c/o Arts Therapies Department
Springfield Hospital
Glenburnie Road
Tooting
London SW17 7DJ
tel: 020 8672 9911

The British Wheel of Yoga
1 Hamilton Place
Boston Road
Sleaford

Lincolnshire NG34 7ES
tel: 01529 306851

Feldenkrais Centre
PO Box 370
London N10 3XA
tel: 020 8346 0258

Gabrielle Roth 5 Rythms
Roland Wilkinson & Susanne
Perks (Second Wave)
Nappers Crossing
Staverton
South Devon TQ9 6PD
tel: 01803 762255
fax: 01803 762255
010522.1732@compuserve.com
messages@onestepbeyond.co.uk

The Laban Centre
(Dance and Movement
Therapy)
Laurie Grove
New Cross
London SE14 6NH
tel: 0208 692 4070
fax: 0208 694 8749
info@laban.co.uk
www.laban.co.uk

LAMAS Qigong
25 Watson road
Worksop
Nottinghamshire S80 2BA
tel: 01909 482 190
fax: 01909 482 156

Moonwan Chi Kung Centre
(London)
tel: 0208 659 0229

Taoist T'ai Chi Centre
Bounstead Road
Blackheath
Colchester
Essex CO2 ODE
tel: 01206 576167
fax: 01206 572269

Tse Qigong Centre
PO Box 116
Manchester M20 3YN
tel: 0161 929 4485

Convergence Therapies

The Bowen Technique
38 Portway
Frome
Somerset BA11 1QU
tel: 01373 461873
bowen@globalnet.co.uk

Metamorphic Association
67 Ritherdon Road
London SW17 8QE
tel: 020 8672 5951
fax: 020 8672 5951
metamorphic@britishisles.
freeserve.co.uk
http://www.geocities.com/
metam

Rosen Method in UK
c/o Ulrika Tham
Neal's Yard Therapy Rooms,
Neal's Yard
Covent Garden
London WC2 9O
tel: 020 7379 7662

The Trager® Association UK
20 Summerdale Road
Hove
East Sussex BN3 8LJ
(for information send an A5 sae)

Zero Balancing Association UK
10 Victoria Grove
Bridport
Dorset DT6 3AA
tel: 01308 420007

Miscellaneous

The Laughter Project
Elms Court
Botley
Oxford OX2 9LP
tel: 01865 244414

Society of Homoeopaths
2 Artizan Road
Northampton
NN1 4HU
tel: 01604 621400
fax: 01604 622622

Body Harmony Institute (UK)
www.bodyharmony.org

Women's Therapy Centre
10 Manor Gardens
London N7 6JS
Advice line: 020 7263 6200

Australia

National Organisations

Australian Complementary
Health Association
247 Flinders Lane
Melbourne 3000
Victoria

Australian Institute of Holistic
Medicine
862 North Lake Road
Jandakot
WA 6164

Australian Natural Therapists
Association
PO Box 856
Coloundra
QLD 4551

Massage Therapies and Aromatherapy

International Federation of
Aromatherapists
1/390 Burwood Road
Hawthorn
VIC 3122

Massage Association of
Australia
PO Box 1187
Camberwell
VIC 3124
info@maa.org.au

Manipulation Therapies and Postural Education

Alexander Technique
International
11 Stanley Street
Darlinghurst
NSW 2010
australia@ati-net.com

Chiropractors' Association of
Australia
459 Great Western Highway
Faulconbridge
NSW 2776
caa-nat@pnc.com.au
Australian Osteopathic
Association
2 Central Avenue
Thornleigh
NSW 2120
aoa@tpgi.com.au

Rolf Institute
Pacific Basin Branch
PO Box 161
Paddington
NSW 2021

Zones, Meridians and Pressure Point Therapies

Australian Acupuncture
Association Ltd
26 Thomas Street
West End
Brisbane
QLD 4810
aaca@eis.net.au

Australian Kinesiology
Association
457 North Road
Ormond 3204

Reflexology Association of
Australia
PO Box 366
Cammeray
NSW 2062

Shiatsu Therapy Association of
Australia
PO Box 1
Balaclava 3183

Metaphysical Therapies

Australian Spiritual Healers
Association
PO Box 4073
Eight Mile Plains
Queensland 4113

Australian Society of Hypnosis
Austin Hospital

Heidelberg
VIC 3084

Movement Therapies

Australian Pilates Method
Association
PO Box 27
Mosman
NSW 2088

Qigong Association of Australia
458 White Horse Road
Surrey Hills
VI 3127

Taoist T'ai Chi Society of
Western Australia
Gregory Street
Geraldton
WA 6530

Australian Institute of Yoga
Therapy
71 Ormond Road
Elwood
VIC 3184
yogather@hotkey.net.au

New Zealand

National Organisations

New Zealand Register of
Complementary Health
Practitioners
c/o New Zealand Health

Network
PO Box 337
Christchurch

Canterbury College of Natural
Medicine
131 Victoria Street
Christchurch

Wellpark College of Natural
Therapies
6 Francis Street
Grey Lynn
Auckland

Manipulation Therapies and Postural Education

New Zealand Chiropractors'
Association
PO Box 7144
Wellesley Street
Auckland

Zones, Meridians and Pressure Point Therapies

New Zealand Reflexology
Association
PO Box 31084
Auckland 9
European Shiatsu School
55 Te Manuao Road
Otaki

Shiatsu Practitioners Association
PO Box 7008
Wellesley Street
Aukland

Metaphysical Therapies

New Zealand Federation of
Spiritual Healers Inc
PO Box 9502
Newmarket
Auckland 1

Reiki New Zealand Inc
PO Box 60-226
Titirangi
Auckland
reiki@ihug.co.nz

USA

National Organisations

American Holistic Medical
Association
6728 Old McLean Village Drive
McLean
VA 223010-3906

American Holistic Health
Association
PO Box 17400
Anaheim
CA 92817-7400
National Association of
Certified Natural Health
Professionals
810 S Buffalo Street
Warsaw
IN 46580

Massage Therapies and Aromatherapy

American Massage Therapy
Association
820 Davis Street
Suite 100
Evanston
IL 60201-4444

Manipulation Therapies and Postural Education

American Chiropractic
Association
1701 Claredon Boulevard
Arlington
VA 22209

American Academy of
Osteopathy
3500 Depauwh Boulevard
Suite 1080
Indianapolis
IN 46268

Alexander Technique Centre
1692 Massachusetts Avenue
Third Floor
Cambridge
MA 02138
Guild for Structural Integration
3107 28th Street
Boulder
CO 80301
gsi@rolfguild.org

Zones, Meridians and Pressure Point Therapies

American Association of
Acupuncture and Bio-Energetic
Medicine
2512 Manoa Road
Honolulu
HI 96822

National Acupuncture
Foundation
1718 M Street
Suite 195
Washington
DC 20036

National Acupuncture and
Oriental Medicine Alliance
14637 Starr Road SE
Olalla
WA 98359

American Oriental Bodywork
Association
6801 Jericho Turnpike
Syosset
NY 11791

School of Shiatsu and Massage
18424 Harbin Springs Road
Middletown
CA 95461

Reflexology Association of
America
4012 South Rainbow Boulevard

PO Box K585
Las Vegas
NV 89103-2059

American Polarity Therapy
Association
2475 Juniper Avenue
Boulder
CO 80301

Metaphysical Therapies

International Association of
Reiki Professionals
PO Box 481
Winchester
MA 01890
info@iarp.org

Sound Healers Association
PO Box 2240
Boulder CO 80306

Body Psychotherapy, Hypnotherapy

The Centre for Energetic
Studies
2045 Fransico Street
Berkeley
CA 94709
http://home.wxs.nl/-
form.psy/home.html

American Institute of
Hypnotherapy
16842 Von Karman Avenue

Apartment 475
Irvine
CA 91724
aih@hypnosis.com

Movement Therapies

American Yoga Association
PO Box 19986
Sarasota
FL 34236

American Dance Therapy
Association
2000 Century Plaza
Suite 108
10632 Little Patuxent Parkway
Columbia
MD 21044-3265

National Qigong (Chi Kung)
Association
571 Selby Avenue
St Paul
MN 55102
webmaster@nqa.org

Feldenkrais Method
3435 Ferry Street
Eugene
Albany
OR 97405
Webmaster@FGNA

Pilates Inc
890 Broadway

Suite 201 6th Floor
New York
NY 10003
Mrpilates@aol.com

Convergence Therapies

Rosen Method
The Berkeley Center
825 Baucroft Way
Berkeley
CA 94710

Trager Institute
21 Locust Avenue
Mill Valley
CA 94941-2806
admin@trager.com

The Metamorphic Technique
Sebastopol
CA

Miscellaneous

Hellerwork International
406 Berry Street
Mount Shasta
CA 96067
hellerwork@hellerwork.com

Academy for Guided Imagery
311 Miller Avenue
Mill Valley
CA 94942

Other Resources: Selected Products for Self-Healing

Audio Cassette: 'Relaxation and Self-Healing, Meditative Exercises to Relax, Revitalise and Ground You' with Kate Williams, tel: 020 8368 9868; fax: 020 8368 8772

CD: 'Opening to Self-Healing, Subtle Energy Exercises and Visualisations – Including Working with the Aura and Chakra System' with Delcia McNeil; tel: 015395 52047 or 020 8442 0391; fax: 015395 52535; delcia.mcneil@virgin.net

For music for healing I recommend Michael Hammer's CDs and audio tapes, available from The School of the Living Light, 47 Aldreth Road, Haddenham, Cambridgeshire CB6 3PW tel: 01353 741760; fax: 01353 741782

High-quality self-help aromatherapy products available from The TLC Collection Ltd, W1V 2LD tel: 01727 874475; fax: 01727 874482 tlc@collection55.freeserve.co.uk; www.tlccollection.com

Biomagnetic products available from Russell McNeil, Independent Supplier, tel/fax: 015395 52535 or tel: 020 8442 0582; russellmcneil.homoeopath@virgin.net

Index

235, 244, 264, 265, 290
insomnia, 82, 96, 124, 131, 183,
    189, 194, 229, 287, 290
intuition, 185, 190, 194, 250, 294
irritable bowel syndrome, 82, 189
isometric and isotonic
    techniques, 76, 299 *n* 6

jade, 195
jasmine, 157, 159, 161
jaw problems, 96
jin shin do, 128, 129
joints structure, 74, 87, 88, 96, 97,
    99, 140, 237, 239, 258, 259,
    261, 268, 290
joy/vitality, 17, 183, 202, 222, 223
Jung, 33, 146, 255, 285
juniper, 82, 158, 160
Jupiter, 160

karma, 21
Keleman, Stanley, 199, 257, 283,
    294
    formative psychology, 257, 294
kinesiology, 33, 54, 139–43, 144
Krieger, Dolores, 167, 168
Kurtz, Ron, 207, 208

labour, 83, 214, 229, 243, 284
lapis lazuli, 159, 160, 195, 196
laughter/laughter therapy, 192,
    226, 253, 257, 289–90
lavender, 80, 82, 84, 85, 160, 161
laying-on hand healing, 97, 167,
    169, 170
learning problems, 90, 271, 272
lemon, 159

light therapy, 290
liver, 157, 183, 189, 191, 196
love, 17, 136, 183, 253, 284, 295
lungs and chest, 158, 159, 183,
    191, 195, 196, 233, 235,
    240, 243, 274, 289
lymphatic system, 69, 75, 90, 125,
    142, 189, 239, 273

ME, 15, 138, 194, 235, 240, 241,
    242, 303, chap10n.7
MS (multiple sclerosis), 15, 240,
    241, 248, 260
magnetic therapy, 275, 290
malachite, 158, 195
manipulation therapies, xvii, 86
marasmus, 41
marjoram, 82
Mars, 158
massage, 13, 14, 16, 18, 26, 40, 44,
    46, 52, 53, 54, 55, 56, 60,
    67–85, 99, 115, 123, 125,
    126, 127, 128, 130, 140,
    142, 169, 211, 213, 214,
    256, 260, 261, 270, 272, 282
McTimoney chiropractic/
    McTimoney, J, 88, 100–101
medical astrology, 289
medical herbalism, xx, 5
meditation, 27, 32, 33, 81, 115,
    128, 129, 134, 135, 149,
    150, 165, 174, 210, 233,
    257, 268, 282, 293, 295
melissa, 159
menopause, 15, 138, 295
menstruation, 23, 117, 128, 131,
    132, 191, 229